The Breuss

Cancer Cure

Rudolf Breuss

books Alive

The Breuss Cancer Cure

Advice for the prevention and natural treatment of cancer, leukemia, and other seemingly incurable diseases

Rudolf Breuss

Note to readers:
The information in this book is for educational purposes only. It is not intended, and should not be considered, as a replacement for consultation, diagnosis or treatment by a duly licensed health practitioner. Anyone who chooses to undertake a therapeutic program is advised to be under the care of a sympathetic and qualified health practitioner.

PUBLISHED BY
Books Alive, a division of Book Pubishing Company
415 Farm Road, Summertown, TN 38483

(931) 964-3571, (888) 260-8458   www.bookpubco.com

Printed in The United States of America

20 19 18 17 16   15 16 17 18 19

Cover design: Ivan A. de Lorenzana   Cover photo: Edmond Fong

Typesetting: Terence Yeung/Peter Virag

Previously published in German by - Eigenverlag Rudolf Breuss
Translated into French, English, Greek, Spanish, Serbian, Croatian, Chinese and Slowanian.

We chose to print this title on responsibly harvested paper stock certified by The Forest Stewardship Council, an independent auditor of responsible forestry practices. For more information, visit https://ic.fsc.org/en

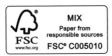

The Library of Congress has already cataloged an earlier printing of the same title under a different publisher name "Alive Books" as follows:
Library of Congress Cataloging-in-Publication Data
Breuss, Rudolf, d. 1991.
   The Breuss cancer cure : advice for the prevention and natural treatment of cancer, leukemia, and other seemingly incurable diseases / Rudolph Breuss.
      p. cm.
Originally published: Burnaby, B.C. : Alive Books, c1995.
Includes bibliographical references and index.
ISBN 978-0-920470-56-5 (alk. paper)
   1. Cancer--Diet therapy. 2. Cancer--Nutritional aspects. 3. Cancer--Alternative treatment. 4. Vegetable juices--Therapeutic use. I. Title.
RC271.D52B73 2007
616.99'40654--dc22   2007033527

To my valued readers and my patients,

I ask you to study my book thoroughly and thoughtfully so that all your doubts are dispelled and your questions are answered.

R. Breuss

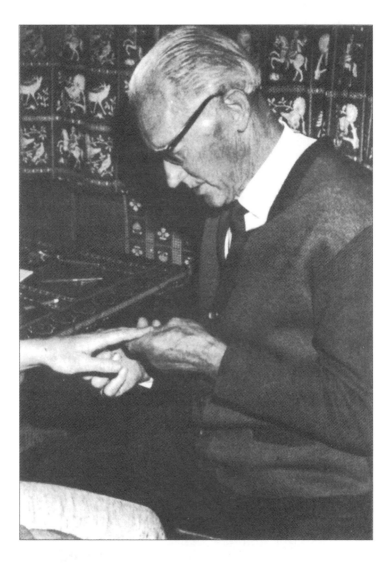

CONTENTS

Foreword   ix

Publisher's Preface   xiii

PART I

Introduction and Testimonial Letters   1

PART II

Can Cancer Be Healed?   19

How the Total Cancer Treatment Works   23

Directions for the Treatment   28

The Correct Way to Follow My Treatment   37

PART III

Treating Leukemia and Other Illnesses   45

Resources   102

List of Herbs   107

Index   109

Foreword

by J. Rancourt, MD

As a medical doctor in Canada, I worked for many years in a special clinic for cancer patients. Everything in the clinic was geared toward making these patients as comfortable as possible until the day they died. It was called palliative care.

At the time I was already using natural healing methods in my private practice. I often thought that there had to be a way of giving these patients a chance for recovery rather than expecting them to die prematurely. Unfortunately, I could not use any alternative methods in the palliative care setting because everything was planned from the perspective of death being inevitable when traditional treatments fail.

Since then, I have gained more and more insight into the nature of chronic disease. I have come to understand that we, as human beings, allow ourselves to become weak, poisoned and ill by moving farther and farther away from the simplicity of nature. We invite chronic illness by greatly disturbing our metabolism through our polluted environment (indoors and out), through our thoughts and attitudes, through our consumption of denatured food and drink and through bad habits such as smoking, drinking and not getting enough rest.

When I first read the book by Rudolf Breuss, which had been presented to me by my colleague, Dr. von Winterfeldt-Schubert, I realized that Breuss' fasting method was the simplest and most natural way possible to treat cancer. Breuss was a humble man whose only desire was to offer help and hope to suffering people. He was so close to the laws of nature that he was able to develop an effective treatment for cancer. His very simplicity gave him an advantage over the complicated and mechanistic way in which medical treatment is often applied today.

Dr. von Winterfeldt-Schubert had learned about the Breuss Treatment at a seminar in Austria in 1986. She was so impressed by it, that she and her husband went on the Breuss fast for three weeks as a means of prevention. During the fast, she continued working and taking courses at the Paracelsus School in Germany. Her husband, an architect, was finishing a large building project for Zaire. Both felt energetic throughout the fast and actually worked harder and better than usual.

The Breuss Treatment is so effective because it deals with cancer and other chronic diseases by cleansing the whole system. The liquids used during the fast are rich in vitamins and minerals, keeping the body nourished; meanwhile, the metabolism is allowed to get back into balance; finally, a deep detoxification process eliminates whatever poisons, abnormalities and wastes are present in the body.

It is vitally important to the success of this treatment that it be followed to the letter. Although people can carry it out by themselves - of course always under a physician's care - the best way to ensure proper fasting is to start out under knowledgeable medical direction. In our experience, the first two weeks of the fast are the most important and, maybe, also the most difficult. After that, the patient has adapted to the fast and will find it easier to return home and finish the treatment even while working again. It is important for the patient to know what is happening inside the body and to learn about proper nutrition to remain fit and healthy after the treatment is over.

A positive outcome of this treatment is closely tied to a person's attitude. People who go through with the six-week fast have a strong will and are convinced and determined that they will heal themselves with natural methods. Since attitude influences the whole metabolism, these people are truly taking their health into their own hands. The fast is often the beginning of a physical and spiritual awakening, compelling people to ensure their future health by turning their lives around, adopting positive habits and living closer to nature.

Once a person has taken the treatment preventively, he will want to repeat it again and again. Dr. von Winterfeldt-Schubert knows people in Germany who fast for two to three weeks every year. Among them is her 83-year-old mother, who is still in perfect health, notwithstanding bearing nine children and surviving two world wars. These people have no Alzheimer's, Parkinson's, arthritis, cancer or any other chronic illnesses. Through repeated preventive fasting such diseases are stopped before they can ever get started.

Dr. von Winterfeldt-Schubert and I are very happy about the new English edition of Rudolf Breuss' book. We believe that this book will give help and hope to many people who previously had no access to his simple, effective treatment.

J. Rancourt, MD
March 27, 1995

Publisher's Preface

Several years ago I received a copy of the German edition of *The Breuss Cancer Cure*. As I started reading, I realized that the author had experienced and was now reporting something phenomenal. I was spellbound. I could not put the book down. I read it in one session. Here, in a very simple way, Breuss was describing how his patients were cured of cancer. They were put on a 42-day juice fast consisting mostly of vegetable juices combined with particular herbal teas. Breuss, a healing practitioner, reported hundreds of cases in which people in his native Austria were cured of cancer and other 'incurable' diseases after taking the 42-day treatment.

In one way, I found this book fascinating reading material; in another way, I was extremely skeptical. My own mother had died of cancer just a few years earlier, and so had many other close friends and relatives. At the time it seemed that once cancer was diagnosed, there was little hope. Each and every person with cancer I had known who had taken conventional treatments with chemotherapy or radiation had neither improved nor survived. It seemed to me that the results of these radical treatments signalled the beginning of the end for the patient. Modern medicine, by its own admission, has not conquered cancer. It has been stuck in a dead-end approach for decades.

Yet here was a man, not even a medical doctor, just a healing practitioner, who was able to cure his patients with a diet of natural juices and herbal teas. *The juice mixture could be prepared at home from organically grown beet roots, carrots, celery roots, black radish and a medium-sized potato.* Later on, Breuss also recommended readily available bottled juices to which lactic acid had been added. Little did Breuss know about the work of the famous German physician, Johannes Kuhl, MD, PhD, who explored the healing effect of lactic acid in the treatment of cancer. Nor was Breuss familiar with the pioneering work of Dr. Lothar Wendt, of Germany, (published as recently as 1989), which connects the protein overload of the cell membrane with all of our degenerative diseases, including cancer. Well before the publication of Wendt's discovery, Breuss put his patients on a juice fast which not only removes the metabolic waste but frees the cell's membrane from the protein build-up which suffocates the cell, preventing proper oxygenation. Knowingly or unknowingly, Breuss administered a program to which modern science and medicine now reluctantly must give credit. Beta-carotene, present in his juice mixture, has now officially been acknowledged as having cancer fighting properties. Enhancing enzymes present in the prescribed juices also contribute a great deal to the success of this juice fast.

Meanwhile, word has spread of many other practitioners treating cancer patients successfully. In Hungary, Dr. Ferenzcy had great success with his red beet juice therapy. Dr. Johanna Budwig, Germany, has successfully used flax oil in combination with quark (a spreadable cheese made from soured milk or buttermilk) to treat cancer patients. Nobel prize laureate Linus Pauling recommended high doses of vitamin C. The Gerson diet includes, amongst other components, a raw food diet of beta-carotene-rich vegetables and a lot of fresh, enzyme rich juices. The treatment of cancer patients with wheat grass juice made Dr. Ann Wigmore world famous. She sparked a revolution which resulted in dozens of so-called 'green' products, such as barley and wheat grass juice powder, appearing on the market. Others have had success in beating cancer with nothing but carrot juice. All of these therapies have one thing in common: they facilitate the oxygenation of the cell.

A number of herbal formulas based on the original formula by Rene Caisse are aimed at treating cancer by removing metabolic waste and inhibiting the growth of the tumor.

Through applying successful observations, and using so-called empirical evidence Rudolf Breuss found a way to help over 6,000 people. I had the privilege of talking to this man while he was still alive. What impressed me most was his humbleness. He told me that he was the object of many attacks by the medical establishment. But his patients were his witnesses. I asked whether he had medical records, X-rays, or any documented evidence of the healing process. He said that the medical doctors had kept such records but were never willing to make them available. Instead, they had denounced his work and often testified that the sick patients that had come to him for help after the doctors had given up on them never had cancer in the first place. Yet cancer had been diagnosed, often by more than one physician, and patients had been told that no more could be done to help them. After undergoing the juice fast and herbal tea treatment, most of these patients lived for more than five years; the medical profession considers a person cured after five years. Breuss gave me permission to phone any of his patients.

The "Total Cancer Treatment," as Rudolf Breuss named his fast, is now offered at a clinic in Hannoversch Münden, Germany. Here patients can fast under medical or clinical supervision. The address and telephone number of this clinic is listed on page 104 of this book.

Cancer, leukemia and other degenerative diseases are of metabolic origin. They are very complex in their manifestations and have numerous causes. Every suggested treatment is only one part in an extremely complex puzzle. It would be irresponsible to say that the Breuss juice fast is the magic bullet that will cure any cancer. Breuss did not invent fasting. People have been fasting throughout recorded history for reasons of health or religion. It is recorded that Jesus fasted for 40 days. Others have fasted even longer. A 42-day fast, as prescribed by Breuss, should present no health problem but should never be embarked upon without medical supervision.

As Dr. Kuhl explains: "The body, fighting for survival, wants to regain its health. It works desperately to reorganize the damaged tissue. To do this it produces the growth substance, lactic acid. But when the level of lactic acid growth becomes toxic, the cells are driven to multiply but not mature. The by-product formed by this struggle is a malignant tumor. The immature cells have failed to develop breathing capacity."

Dr. Kuhl's theory is, in keeping with isopathy, that the cure should fit the disease. "We can help by applying the isopathic principle through the use of small therapeutic quantities of lactic acid. This treatment drains off the pathologically stored lactic acid (D-) inside the body with lactic acid produced by fermentation outside the body (L+) and then administered in therapeutic measure."

Rudolf Breuss makes use of the above principles in his "Total Cancer Treatment."

Just prior to his death on May 17, 1991, at the age of 92, I obtained from Rudolf Breuss the translation rights for an updated version of his original book. It is with much pride that *alive* **books** presents the works of Rudolf Breuss as an educational tool to the English speaking reader.

Siegfried Gursche
Publisher
Vancouver, BC
May, 1995

PART I

Introduction and Testimonial Letters

Laws for the Healer
Who Is Gifted with the Power of Natural Healing

The Bible says, as far as I recall, "He who has been given the power to heal has a God-given gift and should never be mocked, nor has anyone in the world the right to prevent him from healing, or to deprive him of his right to heal." This law, then, is valid throughout the world.

Human beings are so complicated and so different from one another that there is not a physician in the whole world who could say that he can diagnose every illness or always prescribe the right treatment. In my opinion, no medical doctor has the license to claim that only he has the right to help and treat patients. If medical doctors were able to help every patient (which would be marvelous), then, I think, no patient would ever visit a so-called "quack"! Even orthodox physicians visit quacks, naturopaths, non-medical practitioners or homeopaths if they have been very ill and if no other medical doctors or clinics have been able to help them.

A naturopath who only treats patients for money should be classified as a quack – be wary of him. If, however, he only does it to help, he becomes a guide. But if he wants to be a good helper, he must be a good observer and spend a lot of his time studying. A truly dedicated person can learn a great deal, yet no one can help every single person in the world.

A mechanic once said jokingly that he had it a lot harder than a medical doctor because every year there were about 20 new models of cars entering the market, while ever since Adam and Eve, the medical doctor had only two models to deal with! Yet these two models are often such a puzzle and so complicated that so far no one has solved their problems because all of us humans are imperfect.

Who is perfect? Who is like God?

How many people have benefitted from the Breuss treatment? To be on the conservative side, I estimate that up to 1986 about 40,000 patients who had cancer or other seemingly incurable diseases regained their health.

If cancer research organizations and orthodox medicine were with me instead of against me, perhaps the success rate would be in the millions by now.

Even patients who have had operations, radiation treatments or chemotherapy can, in many cases, still benefit from my treatment.

Testimonials and Letters of Thanks

On the following pages, testimonials will be found in the form of letters of thanks from former patients who confirm their healing successes. The original documents are in the hands of the publisher of the original German version of this book.

Intestinal Cancer

December 1, 1971

On July 28, 1964, I was taken into hospital because it was thought I had an obstructed intestine. After a thorough examination the consulting physician diagnosed intestinal cancer. It was suggested that I would have to undergo an operation and have a colostomy.

A short while later my sister Antonie had an inspired vision that I would be healed without having to undergo an operation. I left the hospital and went home. But every day that went by, my condition deteriorated and I knew that I was very close to death.

Then my sister met some acquaintances on a pilgrimage to Wigratzbad, who told her about a gentleman who would treat cancer without performing surgery. My sister asked if they would ask this Mr. Breuss from Bludenz if he could possibly come to her home. He came the very next day and, through eye-diagnosis, confirmed that I had cancer of the large and small intestine. He instructed me to follow his Total Cancer Treatment.

On the 35th day the cancer cleared. Since then I have felt well, have had no complaints and am able to go to work every day.

Many thanks to Our Blessed Lady, the Virgin Mary, who helped me find Mr. Breuss and to Mr. Breuss, whose advice and selfless devotion has aided my complete recovery.

Josef Rädler, 7988 Wangen im Allgäu

Note: Fasting treatment completed in 1964; died on January 8, 1985 of heart failure.

Cancer of the Larynx
December 7, 1972

I shall never be able to thank Mr. Breuss enough for curing me of cancer of the larynx.

For a long time my throat had been very hoarse so I was sent to a throat specialist. The result of the tests showed cancer of the larynx and the doctor advised that I should have an operation immediately. I was thoroughly examined once again and informed that my larynx had to be removed completely. I couldn't decide whether or not to undergo this operation and returned home untreated.

Talking to a neighbor, I heard about a man who had been healed by Mr. Breuss. I went to meet this man who was healthy and happy. He gave me Mr. Breuss' address. I went to see Mr. Breuss personally and he prescribed the juice treatment. By the time I had completed this juice treatment, I felt fit and once again had a good appetite. Despite my 72 years I felt like my old self again.

Thanking you once again for your efforts and your help getting me well again.

Yours faithfully,
Your J. St., 7991 Neukirch

3

Breast Cancer

January 20, 1973

Twenty-three years ago I was supposed to have a breast cancer operation. Despite the fact that year by year my condition was deteriorating, I just couldn't go through with it as my mother had died shortly after undergoing the same kind of operation.

Luckily, five years later, Mr. Breuss was working in our area. I had heard that he was known to heal. I also knew he could diagnose illnesses. I showed him my left hand and asked him, "Am I healthy or ill?" He replied, "Something is not right with your right breast."

I was shocked. Obviously Mr. Breuss hadn't wanted to say it so bluntly because his face reddened. I think maybe he thought that he had said too much.

I then told him not to worry as I already knew that I had breast cancer, but couldn't he possibly do anything for me? He replied, that as I didn't want to undergo an operation and had full knowledge of my illness he had a mixture of juices which he had come up with ten years before, to be used against cancer. Until that day he had never dared mention it to patients who had cancer. As I knew what was wrong with me, he suggested that I follow the juice treatment, even though this particular juice was intended for use against cancer of the stomach. He also warned that I was the first patient he would be testing it on, and that he didn't know if a person could take the treatment for 42 days without having anything else but the juice.

Fully determined, I began the treatment, drinking only the juice. It wasn't easy, because in those days juice extractors had not yet been invented, so I had to grate the vegetables and squeeze out the juices with a towel and potato press.

I was pleasantly surprised. During the treatment I felt very healthy, even though I lost some weight. After 42 days the cancer growth had gone and has never reappeared to this day. I feel very well.

Thank you, Mr. Breuss, from my heart for your advice. I am proud to have been given the chance to be your first patient and to be healed by your juice treatment. I can personally recommend your

Total Cancer Treatment to all cancer sufferers, especially if they have been told no operations can help them.

Maria Nesensohn, Reformhaus (Health Food Store)
Gartenstrasse 15, 6700 Bludenz

Note: Still healthy, January 1986.

Pinched Nerve
January 20, 1973

A few years after you had healed me of breast cancer by prescribing the Total Cancer Treatment, I suddenly got very bad headaches and thought that I had developed a brain tumor. Obviously I was shocked, so once again, I contacted you, Mr. Breuss, for an eye diagnosis. Fortunately you diagnosed that I did not have a tumor but a pinched nerve between the third and fourth cervical vertebrae. You sent me to a chiropractor in Zürich. My husband and I told this medical doctor your diagnosis and he X-rayed me. He confirmed your diagnosis and was amazed because in his field he had never come across anyone who could diagnose a case like this so accurately.

We explained to him that this excellent diagnostician was an electromechanic who, apart from his work, was interested in natural healing and was happy to help sick people. To which he replied that he had a high regard for this man.

After several treatments by this chiropractor in Zürich my headaches disappeared.

Once again, Mr. Breuss, I would like to thank you for your diagnosis and the good advice you have again so selflessly given to me.

Yours gratefully,
Maria Nesensohn, Reformhaus (Health Food store)
Gartenstrasse 15, 6700 Bludenz

Note: Mrs. Nesensohn is still running her shop – January 1986.

Kidney Cancer
January 23, 1973

On February 12, 1970, my family doctor sent me to a university hospital. They carried out tests and the result showed that I had a tumor on my left kidney. Once this was found, they carried out further procedures to find the exact position of the tumor.

On March 3, 1970, I was sent to the hospital. I had an operation on March 5, 1970, to remove the kidney with a large tumor on it which turned out to be malignant (cancer).

I was sent home on March 17, 1970. My husband was asked to see the surgeon and was informed that I had only one year to live. At home, my treatment was taken over by my family doctor and a radiologist. I got 43 radiation treatments and had to go for an X-ray every three months.

On September 9, 1971, I was in the hospital once again because X-rays had found a tumor on my left lung. I underwent another operation during which the left pulmonary lobe was removed. I was discharged from the hospital on October 8, but had to continue medical supervision. In May 1972 the X-rays showed that I had another tumor on my right lung. Another operation was advised, but I refused.

By a divine miracle I got the address of a man who could heal cancer. I drove immediately to see Mr. Breuss in Thüringerberg, Austria.

Mr. Breuss confirmed my cancer but raised my hopes by telling me that in 42 days I would be completely healed if I followed his Total Cancer Treatment. Even though I was still under my family doctor's and radiologist's care, I began the treatment. After four weeks of Mr. Breuss' treatment I had to visit the radiologist again, who confirmed that the tumor was now only the size of a small rice corn. As I ended the treatment after a further four weeks, I had to visit the radiologist once again. All that could be seen was a scar. This was all medically confirmed.

I cannot thank Mr. Breuss enough for curing me of my "incurable" disease. I am convinced that if I had known about him earlier, I would not have had to undergo the pain and suffering of the previous operations.

M.H., 7990 Friedrichshafen

Note: This lady still feels very well in 1986.

Lump in the Breast

February 7, 1973

On September 19, 1972, I discovered a large hard lump in my right breast. My family doctor checked me into the hospital immediately to have surgery. I had already heard about the Breuss juice treatment and decided to try it before agreeing to the operation. After three weeks of the juice treatment the growth began to change and after six weeks of the treatment it had completely disappeared. My doctor was amazed and told me that the growth was so large that I would have undergone a complete mastectomy.

I am very happy about my successful treatment because I am only 40 years old and can now go on living a normal life.

To Mr. Breuss who has already helped many people with his treatment and to our Lord I would like to say thank you. I can only hope that Mr. Breuss will continue to help me and many other patients for many years to come.

Mrs. G.S., 7988 Wangen im Allgäu

Note: 1985, everything is still excellent.

Leukemia, Arthritis, Myocarditis

[undated]

Christmas 1964 I became ill with leukemia, arthritis and myocarditis. I was sent to the hospital and my condition wasn't getting any better until my husband brought Mr. Breuss to see me in the hospital. Mr. Breuss had already commented to my husband, while on their way from Wigratzbad to Ravensburg, that I would feel much better after three days and would be allowed home after six days. I drank the tea and juice and, very soon, I was feeling a lot better. After approximately six days I was discharged from hospital. I am extremely thankful to Mr. Breuss for his time and treatment.

Mrs. Pia H., 7989 Argenbühl

Liver and Pancreas Problems

1974

My history of illnesses is probably typical of of what many patients go through.

For years I had liver and pancreas disease and had never found any treatment that made it better, even though I consulted various medical doctors. I was kept on a strict diet and had to take a lot of medicines to just keep the disease at bay, though I could only do this to a certain degree.

A while later, I also got kidney disease. In short, my state of health had arrived at the zero mark.

One day a friend of mine gave me Mr. Breuss' address. As I had nothing to lose, I drove to Thüringerberg immediately.

Without even being told about my history of illnesses he confirmed the medical doctor's diagnosis. He prescribed a juice treatment for six weeks and I did exactly as prescribed. During this time it was quite unpleasant, but I stuck it out. It was worth it in the end.

Now I feel healthy and can eat everything and I don't suffer even the slightest symptoms of my former disease.

I can recommend this treatment as, once again, I am a happy and content human being.

Yours faithfully,
X.H., 7992 Tettnang

Cancer of the Lip

[undated]

During May 1971 I had an operation on my lower lip. A medical evaluation from a university clinic then confirmed that I had cancer. Consequently, I received 25 radiation treatments.

In 1973 the cancer came back. Radiation couldn't help anymore. In the spring of 1974 I was sent to the university clinic again to undergo a major operation and to have plastic surgery involving skin transplants. The plan was to do five transplants, each a year apart. I have to mention that, in addition, I had three lumps in my glands and throat, which were confirmed to be 100 per cent cancerous.

My operation was scheduled for March 29, 1974 at 10 a.m. At 7:30 a.m. that morning I telephoned the medical doctor and told him that I had decided not to undergo the operation (after which I would have had to spend a whole year in the hospital). He unwillingly discharged me and told me that I alone was responsible for the outcome of that decision.

When I returned home, my wife and I drove to Bludenz to Mr. Breuss who prescribed the Total Cancer Treatment, which I started the very next day.

I felt very well during the treatment. After four weeks we began to see results. Five weeks later my lip had healed and the lumps had completely disappeared. One week after the treatment I started work again. I had never felt so well and I still feel the same way now.

Therefore, I cannot thank Mr. Breuss enough.

Yours faithfully,
Peter Seehuber, Isny/Allgäu

Blood Poisoning
May 20, 1974

In 1938 I had very bad blood poisoning in my left arm. It was very swollen and colored blue, red and green. I had to go to the medical doctor who took one look at it and said it was too late, there was nothing more they could do for me.

Mr. Breuss offered me his help. What he did was a natural miracle. A short while later I could go swimming. I would like to thank Mr. Breuss for saving my life.

Emil Siess, 6714 Nüziders, Tänzerweg 8

Damaged Disc
September 1, 1974

For years I had suffered from backache (damaged disc). On June 30, 1974, Mr. Rudolf Breuss visited us and painlessly eased the dislocated disc back into place. After this manipulation, the pain was gone and now, two months later, it still has not recurred.

I am very grateful to Mr. Breuss and would suggest this painless and benign treatment to any patient.

E.N. Friedrichshafen

Damaged Disc

October 16, 1974

You will probably remember that on November 18th, 1972, I consulted you regarding treatment of my damaged disc.

I can now confirm that you have helped me to an almost unbelievable degree. As you know, I am an enthusiastic skier and always had back problems when pursuing this sport. Two years have passed and to this day I have had no recurrences. I should also mention that your treatment healed me almost immediately.

I must admit that I was very skeptical of your treatment at first; therefore, I have only written now, two years later, because your treatment has now been proven. It worked!
For two years I have not suffered from any back pains.

I would like to thank you for your care and remain,

Yours gratefully,
Albert Bildstein, Professor
High School, Feldkirch, Austria

Stomach Problems

February 20, 1975

My mother, Mrs. Sofie Wachter, Bludenz, became so seriously ill on January 6, 1963, that three medical doctors were consulted. For five whole weeks she brought up everything she ate or drank, which was very little, only tea and rusks.

As she brought the food up again it was heavily mixed with blood. The doctors thought that she had cancer, but also that there was a possibility that she had an abscess of the pancreas. My mother's condition was so bad that she could not be moved; therefore, she could not have an X-ray. Thus, they diagnosed the two possibilities merely by her symptoms. In any case, the doctors had completely given up on her, since, according to them, both illnesses would be fatal.

As a last resort, I contacted Mr. Breuss in Bludenz who prescribed a juice of beet roots, carrots and celery root (celeriac). We followed exactly as prescribed by Mr. Breuss' instructions. After a week we saw a small improvement – at least she wasn't bringing everything up again. Slowly it stopped completely and we could see even more improvement. Four months later, to the surprise of the medical doctors, she was healed.

Every year, without fail, we follow this juice therapy for my mother and after this treatment she always feels healthy, especially her heart. My mother is still alive and now in her 88th year. We would like to thank you once again for everything you have done.

K.L., Bludenz, Vorarlberg

Note: At 88 years old, Frau Wachter still did her daily housework.

Abdominal Cancer

April 30, 1975

During 1962 and 1966 I underwent surgery and also eight weeks of radiation therapy with liquid radioactive gold injected under my abdominal wall. Until the summer of 1967, my condition had been quickly deteriorating. Another blood test had shown a new invasion of cancerous cells. I sensed that my body was shutting down more and more. When I heard about people who had been healed trying the "juice treatment," I went to visit Mr. Breuss. He examined my eyes and suggested that I start his juice treatment right away. As I could rest a lot and lived in a wooded area where I could enjoy the fresh air, it was easier not to feel too hungry during my weeks of fasting. Only in the last five days did I have an additional half cup of gruel twice a day.

I firmly believe that during this treatment my blood renewed itself and enabled me to overcome this disease. I still have some pain which I attribute to radiation, to adhesions and to the radioactive gold.

During the juice treatment my tongue went completely black. I consulted Mr. Breuss who suggested drinking pimpernel root tea to clear my tongue, rather than ceasing the juice diet. Indeed, within three weeks complete recovery took place!

T.S. 7988 Wangen im Allgäu

Note: This lady still feels well in 1986.

Cancer of the Stomach and Intestines

August 18, 1975

Twenty-five years ago I was diagnosed with cancer of the stomach and intestines. I was supposed to have surgery but could not make up my mind. Then I had a chance meeting with a gentleman from Bludenz, Mr. Breuss, who was visiting a cancer patient in Götzis. Mr. Breuss told me about his Total Cancer Treatment and I decided immediately to do this juice treatment together with Mr. Josef Fend who had stomach cancer.

After 42 days the cancer discharged itself through the bowels and the same thing happened on the same day to Mr. Josef Fend. After the treatment, the X-rays showed no sign of cancer. To this day there have been no recurrences. During the treatment I lost about 15 kg (33 lbs). I was the third person to try Mr. Breuss' treatment and would recommend it to anyone. I cannot thank you enough, Mr. Breuss, for all you have done.

The treatment wasn't easy to follow because at that time we did not have juice presses – but the result was worth both the trouble and the patience required.

Olga Marte, 6840 Götzis

Note: Now, in 1986, Mrs. Marte is still in excellent health.

Breast Cancer

Fall 1977

After a diagnosis of breast cancer (right side), I followed the Total Cancer Treatment in July and August, 1977.

Result: The hardened area returned to normal.

My state of health as of today: excellent.

Remarks: An amazing improvement of the blood (formation and structure of the red blood cells) during the Breuss Total Cancer Treatment.

H.S., CH-8580 Amriswil/Switzerland

Note: Still in very good health in 1986.

Cancer/Slipped Disc
October 11, 1979

In the autumn of 1966 I was diagnosed with cancer, so I tried the Total Cancer Treatment.

Condition of health to this day: no recurrence (1979).

After the treatment I felt like a new-born baby!

Besides that, for years I had a slipped disc so I could barely bend down. After only one treatment from Mr. Breuss, this condition was alleviated and I have never suffered from it again.

I cannot thank Mr. Breuss enough.

P.H., Wangen im Allgäu

Hardened Mammary Glands
November 19, 1979

Dear Mr. Breuss,

Because of hardened mammary glands and a suspicion of cancer, it was suggested in August (of this year) that I undergo a complete mastectomy. At the suggestion of Hans Neuner I tried many poultices and additional extracts and teas. My condition improved slightly until suddenly I felt a large gland under my armpit. Surgery seemed unavoidable.

It must have been a miracle that I suddenly came across your book. I decided at once to try your Total Cancer Treatment, even though I was severely underweight (45 to 55kg) [99 to 121 lbs].

Now I have made it through 38 days without needing gruel, and I hope to continue this well during the remaining four days. The lumps have shrunk significantly and the gland in my armpit has receded. I thank God for this miracle!

To you my sincere thanks for passing on your knowledge and experience, all that you have discovered and researched during many decades of difficult work.

Once again, many thanks,
H.G., A 5431 Kuchl/Salzburg

Lupus

March 6, 1980

There is a miraculous person in Bludenz whose name is Mr. Breuss. I would like to thank you a thousand times for your outstanding abilities. No medical doctor would have been able to heal my lupus. I was 27 years young when I received a written diagnosis from Dr. Kiedermair of Linz which said "incurable". So, as a last resort, I drove to Mr. Zeileis in Gallspach, who said, "I can try and restrain the disease but am not able to heal it." Twelve times I went through his treatment. And now, at 66, a new god appeared who suggested the juice and tea treatment which healed me. Mr. Breuss, I feel like hugging and kissing you.

My six-week-long treatment finished in December. I did not write straight away in case there were any side effects, but during the treatment I felt fantastic, and in thankfulness, I am remaining faithful to the juice and continue to drink 1/4 liter every day. I would recommend to everyone to do the same as myself and thousands of other people. I only hope, Mr. Breuss, that as a reward for your healing method, you will live a long, happy and healthy life.

Yours faithfully,
R.D., 4020 Linz/D.

Breast Cancer

March 12, 1980

After being diagnosed with cancer of the breast, I started the Total Cancer Treatment on October 25, 1977.

The result was very good.

My state of health now, on December 3, 1980, is still good.

Further comments: none.

Z.H. A. 3340 Waidhofen a/d. Ybbs

Uterine Cancer

December 28, 1981

Diagnosis: Uterine Cancer

Total Cancer Treatment taken: September 14 to October 26, 1981

Result: Good

State of Health: Good

I have never felt as good as after this treatment. Blood pressure, blood sugar and blood count were all better than they had been in years of taking medication. In January, I will do a second treatment, which I recommend to anyone. During the fast I was so fit that I could do all my work with ease. Dear Mr. Breuss, I am grateful to you from the bottom of my heart, and I hope that you will be able to help many more poor sick people with your Total Cancer Treatment.

Elfriede Sommer

A-8052 Graz-Wetzelsdorf

Note: I received written Christmas greetings from Mrs. Elfriede Sommer on December 14, 1985.

Hodgkin's Disease

February 27, 1977

Dear Mr Breuss,

You will probably remember that at the beginning of January 1977 my husband and I travelled from Lucerne (Switzerland) to consult with you. At that time I had suffered from Hodgkin's disease for more than eight years and doctors had finally told me that I would not live beyond the middle of April. By chance I read about your healing successes in our local newspaper. You advised me to take the Total Cancer Treatment, which I started immediately following our visit. I followed the treatment strictly for two weeks, after which I ate normally but continued to take the teas and juice mixture. In the fourth week I went to my doctor for a blood test. My doctor, by the way, was angry with me because I had stopped taking my medication. After looking at the test results, he shook my hand and said he wanted to congratulate me because my blood looked so good that it could not be any better. In three weeks my blood volume had increased by twenty per cent and the blood itself looked so good that he could only advise me to continue the juice treatment. I feel better now than I have felt in years. Even after the treatment I am still drinking a glass of the juice and the sage tea every day.

I don't know how to thank you for saving my life. Could you send me about ten copies of your little book? There is great demand for it.

I have one more big favor to ask. My mother has been suffering from multiple sclerosis for fifteen years and has been in a wheelchair for the past five years. Mentally, she is completely fit. Is there a possibility for improvement? Please answer me as soon as possible.

Once again, many many thanks.

Mrs. Silvia Martina

CH-6014 Littau

Hodgkin's Disease - *continued*

September 6, 1982

Dear Mr. Breuss,

Maybe you will remember that six years ago I came to you with an advanced state of Hodgkin's disease. I am doing extremely well today and my doctors are still amazed. My family doctor declared last week that I was the only patient he knew who had survived this disease. I am enclosing a more official statement which will please you, I think, because you have spent so many years trying to cure different diseases with natural juices and teas.

I hope you are well; after all these years I would like to thank you again from my heart. May you stay happy and healthy and enjoy your great successes for many more years.

With best wishes,

S.M. (Silvia Martina)

Hodgkin's Disease - *continued*
(Silvia Martina's official statement)

September 6, 1982

Six years ago doctors confirmed that I was in the advanced stages of lymphatic cancer and that I had only three months to live. I have a family with two daughters, and I was thirty years old at the time. It was about the worst thing that could have happened to me. The medical treatment, the injections, were excruciating; I was reduced to nothing but sickness and suffering, and all that pain was merely serving to prolong a hopeless life for a few more months. At that point I heard about Mr. Breuss from people who had already had good results with the juice treatment. My husband and I went to him immediately and Mr. Breuss advised me to try the juice treatment, but without taking medications, if possible. I told my doctors that I would stop my medications, to which they replied whether I was aware that this was a matter of life and death. I started the juice and tea treatment at once. After four weeks I went to my doctor for a blood test. After the test I went home laughing and crying. The blood test was better than any other. My blood volume had increased to a level of eighty per cent. I feel healthier now than ever before. All this is now six years past. I still go for a blood test every three months and have been getting the same good results with every one of them. All the doctors tell me that I am living a second life. Ever since taking the treatment, I have been drinking sage tea every day and I will continue drinking it always.

To Mr. Breuss, who saved my life in his simple and humble way, I would like to express my deep-felt gratitude once again.

Silvia Martina

Headaches

January 20, 1985

About 24 years ago, during gym class at school, I fell down flat and was knocked unconscious for a short time. Because of this fall, I suffered severe headaches and could hardly sleep at night. I had to have a spinal tap at the hospital and the doctor suggested an operation to insert a silver plate in my skull. I refused to undergo this procedure. Then some people whom Breuss had already helped suggested that I contact him. When I saw him, he did an eye diagnosis and recommended his juice treatment. I noticed a positive effect after only a few days. I was able to sleep again and after the treatment, that is, after 42 days, I had regained my full health. Since then, I have had no recurrences. I really admire Mr. Breuss and am extremely grateful that he has helped me to regain my health.

A.M., Prof. Dr. M.A.

Altach, Egethen 6

Damaged Discs

January 20, 1985

Fifteen years ago I suffered from badly damaged discs. In the Kneipp Club of Götzis Mr. Breuss gave a talk bout the topic "Disc Problems." I took a treatment from him and he delivered me from my serious suffering. I remain grateful to Mr. Breuss to this day. I would like to add that I was privileged to be the first person to experience his painless manipulation.

H.E.

Götzis

Back Problems

January 20, 1985

I am, or was, a mail carrier. For six years I had suffered from disc problems and bone deterioration. I could barely walk fifty meters without collapsing.

By chance I got to know Mr. Breuss. He eased my discs back into place, and since then I have been free from pain. For six years I had visited every doctor who had been recommended to me as being excellent, but all in vain.

For the rest of my life I will thank this wonderful man who wants nothing more in this world than to help other people. I hope that Mr. Breuss will live among us for many more healthy years.

With many thanks for everything,

E.A.

Götzis, Romerweg 23

PART II

Can Cancer Be Healed?

Cancer develops in people primarily through a certain predisposition and the combined effect of repeated assaults of carcinogens on the system. Longtime exposure to even small amounts of carcinogens can damage one's health; if this damage is ignored and not treated, it can lead to cancer. Oftentimes carcinogens enter our food supply by way of processing and preservation methods, such as adding artificial color or overheating food.

The following nine warning signs should be noted:
1. Palpable lumps or hardening, especially in the breasts.
2. Noticeable changes on nipples or in birth marks.
3. Persistent changes in bowel habits or urination.
4. Persistent sore throats or coughs.
5. Difficulty swallowing at an older age.
6. Heavy bleeding or prolonged discharge from any natural body opening. Also bleeding outside the normal menstrual cycle.
7. Wounds that will not heal.
8. Swellings which do not recede.
9. Noticeable weight losses or gains (not based on dieting, fasting or continuous overeating.)

I do not mean to alarm you or to say that any of the above conditions will necessarily indicate cancer. On the contrary, it is far more likely that these changes mean something else, because many illnesses show similar symptoms and other diseases are, after all, far more frequent than cancer. But if you notice any of the above signs, you should immediately go for a check-up and for prevention follow my Total Cancer Treatment as soon as possible.

Most Frequent Cancers

The main cause of throat and lung cancer is smoking. A smoker is 20 times more susceptible to lung cancer than someone who does not smoke. Therefore, please do not smoke and try your best to prevent your children from ever developing this evil habit.

Cancer of the womb (uterine cancer) starts with no symptoms and without any pain. Signs could be irregular bleeding, especially during menopause. In younger women watch out for irregular bleeding, or bleeding between periods or following sexual intercourse. Another sign to watch for is bleeding after urinating, after relieving the bowels or after very strenuous work. Left untreated, cancer of the womb will lead to death. However, if immediately after symptoms appear you start the Total Cancer Treatment and take the prescribed teas you can be healed.

Breast cancer develops very gradually. Hardening, lumps, or shrinkage in the breasts could be early signs of cancer developing. Pain and ulceration usually only appear when the cancer is in its advanced stages.

Suggestions for Prevention:

1. Take care to exercise regularly to keep your body fit.
2. Breathe deeply in clean, fresh air.
3. Avoid smoky and stale air.
4. Do not smoke.
5. Favor natural and vitamin-rich nutrition.
6. Avoid overeating.
7. Always maintain regular digestion, and correct irregularities immediately to avoid greater problems.
8. Last but not least: do not be afraid of cancer! Fear is your worst enemy.

What Is a Cancerous Growth or Tumor?

A cancerous tumor is an independent growth that is mainly caused by pressure. If, for example, a patient has been suffering from stomach trouble for several years and food stays in his stomach for hours on end, it produces pressure on the stomach glands and wall, which can then lead to cancer of the stomach. Many years ago, I knew a man who, from early evening to late at night, smoked a long pipe and always placed it on the same side of his mouth. I once said to his wife that her husband would definitely get lip cancer. After approximately 10 years, his wife approached me and asked me to go and see her husband. I asked, "Why, has he got lip cancer?" His wife looked surprised and replied, "Yes, how did you know?" I then reminded her that I had warned her 10 years earlier.

Because of prolonged unnatural pressure on a certain part of the body, no blood flows to this spot so that it would normally die. However, this pressure point wants to live, too, and so it defends itself by drawing and sucking missing materials from its surroundings. Through this independent suction, in my opinion, an independent growth is formed.

In the beginning this entity grows very slowly, and it often takes, as you know, 10 or more years, until it suddenly grows very quickly into what we call cancer. When the cancer has reached that stage it is high time (but not too late by far) to start the Total Cancer Treatment. If, at the very beginning, one cuts into or presses around such a harmless and small growth (i.e. early detection), then it becomes wild, because the cancer then enters the bloodstream, giving rise to metastasis. It is better not to disturb a lump or growth. Instead, another treatment is required.

How Can Cancer Be Treated?

"How can this treatment be carried out?" I often thought.

Then the idea came to me that it would be possible to help with vegetable juices. It was a discussion on the subject with a prominent member of the Kneipp therapy movement, Mr. Balestrang, which gave me the idea.

I combined a number of vegetable juices into one mixture as outlined in my Total Cancer Treatment. I thought out my vegetable juice treatment as follows: Red beet root juice is definitely helpful against cancerous growths, but it is impossible to live on red beet juice alone. So I added carrots because of the carotene, celeriac because of its phosphorus content – without phosphorus we cannot survive – and black radish and potato for the liver.

Since 1950, I have helped many hundreds of people with different types of cancer and leukemia whom the medical profession had given up, as apparent from the letters of thanks that I received.

When you read my Total Cancer Treatment you will probably think what many patients and medical doctors have thought and said: "It is impossible to live on nothing but juice for 42 days." Many doctors have written to me saying that it is impossible to live for that length of time with no fat or protein and that they did not want to take the responsibility for this juice fast. I always gave the same answer: You cannot take the responsibility for giving the patients something to eat. The only patients that died were patients that were given something to eat. I have had thousands of experiences with the effects of my treatment and have convinced medical doctors who had their doubts.

Many medical doctors have said to my patients that they did not believe in my treatment but were surprised by my successes and thereafter were in favor of it. I think these professional doctors with their objective attitudes deserve the highest respect.

How the Total Cancer Treatment Works

Over time I have learned from experience. It used to puzzle me why cancer patients who only had a small cancerous growth or who had already been operated on could only barely manage or not manage at all without eating during the juice treatment. The following report will help to throw some light on this riddle.

In 1962 I visited a woman who had incurable cancer of the stomach. For one and a half months, this woman had drunk and eaten next to nothing but had been vomiting daily. You will think that is impossible. I said at that time that this woman had lived on her cancerous growth for that period. Every morning and evening I gave her three tormentil (*Tormentilla erecta*) tincture drops on her tongue because she could not swallow the tormentil tea. I gave her these drops to close the ulcerated cancer cells, which I succeeded in doing. By the third day she ceased vomiting and was able to take two tablespoons of vegetable juice. Every day she began to take more. On the 10th day her doctor, who had visited her daily, said to her, "Well, you certainly have improved a lot." He asked the woman, "Are you able to eat anything?" to which she answered, "Yes." He asked: "What can you eat?" She replied, "Only juices." He asked, "And that keeps you settled? Don't you have to vomit any more?" She replied,"No."

During the course of the treatment she used very little juice.

It is now clear to me why patients suffering from a large tumor only drink a little juice and need not eat in between. They do not require any protein. On the other hand, those who have only a small growth (in the early stages) find it hard to live on only vegetable juices. In such cases one half cup of clear onion broth per day is allowed, as there is a need for protein. (See recipe at the

23

end of Directions for the Treatment, in Part II.) That also applies to cancer patients who have undergone surgery with partial or complete tumor removal.

Bruno Vonarburg, the writer of the book *God's Blessing on Nature*, (Christian Books), confirms the following about my Total Cancer Treatment:

> Because the development of the carcinogenic process, that is the degeneration of the growth and tumorous proliferation, is being fed by protein, I see the following advantages for the application of the juice treatment:

> During this treatment protein intake is stopped, because there is no protein in the daily diet. But since the organism is unable to live without protein, the protein-starved blood cells attack everything nonessential, such as growths, waste matter and boils. *This is akin to an operation without a knife*, which the white blood corpuscles accomplish meticulously.

> Secondly, another most important element lies in the rich mineral content of the vegetable juices. It can be proven that when cancer attacks the body, the mineral balance in the body cells is disturbed and the mineral-rich vegetable juices can positively influence and counterbalance this mineral disturbance.

> During the juice treatment it is, of course, important to expel urine and stool regularly, so that the waste products do not stay in the body too long and poison the organism. The organs of excretion will be helped to work by the daily tea combination. Cranesbill tea stimulates the kidneys to excrete poisons and to cleanse the blood, while sage tea stops infection. Marigold tea suppresses the so-called "viromycose," i.e. eliminates disturbances of the cellular respiration processes. In other words, the complete juice therapy must be viewed within this triple effectiveness."

I would like to add that many people not suffering from cancer have also tried my juice treatment, some to prevent illness, others to lose weight. These people have felt well and were able to work even without supplementary eating. Remember that the juices contain no protein, a good indication that the body can manage without protein replacement for quite some time. Hopefully, after I have explained all this, there will be no questions left unanswered.

A Few Examples

In 1950, a woman who had for a long time suffered from breast cancer was the very first patient who tried my juice treatment. She recovered and is still healthy today, in 1986, and there is no sign of any tumor (refer to *Testimonials*). I had already formulated my juice treatment ten years before that, but in those days never dared to tell any of my patients that they suffered from cancer.

This particular lady had known for a long time that she had cancer because she was supposed to have surgery but could not make the decision because her mother, suffering also from breast cancer, had been operated on and had died shortly afterwards. At the time I said to this lady, "If you know what you suffer from, I have a remedy, but I have only studied it with cancer of the stomach."

I suggested she try it as it could not do her any harm. It was not an easy undertaking because there were no juicers in those days. The vegetables had to be grated through a vegetable shredder and afterwards pressed with a ricer [potato press] or squeezed out with a linen towel.

This lady, Mrs. M.N. of Bludenz, was healed after 42 days with no signs of the tumor left.

My second case: After treating this woman from Bludenz, I was asked to visit a Mr. Josef F. in Götzis who suffered from cancer of the stomach. He was inoperable and given no hope for recovery. He also tried my Total Cancer Treatment and after 42 days he was well again. He only died in 1971 at the age of 80.

I also visited Mrs. Olga M. in Götzis who suffered from stomach and intestinal cancer. She also tried my juice treatment (together with Mr. Josef F.) and after 42 days, she, too, was healed and is still alive and well today (1986)!

My fourth case was Sister Leonarda von Zams who suffered from intestinal cancer. She followed my Total Cancer Treatment and was also healed. At the age of 80, she was still able to continue working as an artist.

More and more patients began to come to me and on July 28, 1964, I was asked to go to the Sanitarium Maria vom Sieg in Wigratzbad near Wangen im Allgäu. Mr. Josef Rädler, the brother of Miss Antonie Rädler, the owner of the health clinic, was suffering from cancer of the large and small intestines. He was considered a terminal case. They still wanted to operate on him (colostomy), but with the knowledge that "if he isn't operated on he will die soon and if he is operated on he will not live much longer, either."

Miss Rädler then got an "inspiration from above," as she called it, that her brother would recover without undergoing an operation if he promised to say the rosary every day of his life with his whole family. However, should he undergo an operation, he would die.

She then took her brother out of the hospital, just before the surgery. Nothing happened except that Mr. Rädler's condition became worse day by day and his wife and relatives were becoming desperate. After 10 days, a Mr. A.S. from Bludenz was visiting and Miss Rädler told him about her anguish. He told her of a man in Bludenz who had completely healed a 70-year-old woman suffering from terminal cancer of the stomach, a completely hopeless case. "As a last resort, this man, Mr. Breuss, was called and she fully recovered. "

To this Miss Rädler said, "Then maybe he will be able to help my brother as well. Would it be possible to telephone Mr. Breuss and ask him to come?"

I then spoke to Miss Rädler on the telephone and she asked if I could come immediately. I didn't want to go. But when she told me that her brother had eight children and that the youngest was only two years old, I could not decline. I went the very next day, July 28, 1964, taking my wife along.

It was 11:55 a.m. when I examined Mr. J. Rädler who was in his office on a stretcher. By examining his eyes, I diagnosed that he was suffering from cancer of the large and small intestines. Miss

Rädler told me that it was exactly the same diagnosis as the hospital's. The eight children then began to cry. I told them that if I could not help, I would not say anything in front of the patient. I added that he had a very healthy heart and strong lungs and would be able to easily withstand my juice treatment and would definitely be able to work again (which he was able to) as you can see in his letter of thanks (See Introduction and Testimonial Letters, in Part I.), Mr. Rädler was still capable of work in his late seventies. He died 20 years after his recovery, on January 1, 1985.

Because of Mr. Rädler, many thousands of patients came to visit me with various ailments, especially patients suffering from cancer and leukemia. Most of the ones who suffered from terminal illnesses became healthy again. I repeat – do not be frightened by cancer and leukemia any more.

Directions for the Treatment

With this treatment the patient is not allowed to eat at all for 42 days other than taking the vegetable juices and teas recommended. The juices can be taken only in the amounts stated. They can be taken as much as required for hunger, though not in excess of one half liter (2 cups/500 ml) per day. The less juice the patient drinks the better.

It is possible, and in a way preferable, to make the juice at home, if you can obtain organically grown vegetables.

If this is not the case or if you do not want to take the trouble, most health food stores offer the organic "Breuss Vegetable Juice Mix" which is prepared by a Swiss company under my directions.

My Juice Mixture:

To prepare the juice, take 3/5 beets, 1/5 carrots, 1/5 celeriac, and then add a little black radish and one egg-sized potato. For example:

300 g (9.6 oz.) beet root
100 g (3.2 oz.) carrots
100 g (3.2 oz.) celeriac (celery root)
30 g (1.06 oz.) black radish juice
1 potato, the size of an egg

Note: It is not crucial to add the potato juice, except for cancer of the liver where it is absolutely necessary. Instead of adding the potato to the juice mixture, you can drink a cup of potato peel tea each day. This tea is to be slowly sipped cold. To prepare the tea, take a handful of potato peelings in one cup of water and boil for two to four minutes. If this tea does not taste good, then your liver does not need it, so you do not have to drink it.

Use a modern juice extractor, or press the vegetables the old-fashioned way, then put the juices through a tea strainer or a linen towel. There is a tablespoon of sediment for each quarter liter of juice which must not be consumed. This sediment would make the juice more difficult to drink and, more importantly, would serve as food for the cancer.

The cancer lives only on solid foods taken into the body. If for 42 days the patient only drinks vegetable juices and tea, the cancerous growth dies while the person can live through it all very well!

During this time the patient may lose 5 to 15 kg (11 to 33 lbs) but will feel quite well during the treatment period. I myself have tried this treatment and was able to work harder than ever before. It is better if a few days before starting this treatment, the patient drinks approximately one quarter liter (1 cup/250 ml) of juice per day. The patient may go up to one half liter but this is not necessary.

Drink the juice slowly with the help of a spoon. Do not swallow it immediately but let the juice remain in the mouth for a few moments. Every now and again the patient may have a mouthful of sauerkraut juice which is beneficial to the patient.

Important Teas for Cancer Treatment

1. Sage Tea

For gargling, the sage herb (*Salvia officinalis*) should be steeped in hot water for ten minutes, but to drink it, the herb must be boiled for exactly three minutes. Place one, at the most two, teaspoons of sage in one half liter (2 cups/500ml) of boiling water. Boil for three minutes, then let cool. Sage contains a large amount of essential oils, which are very important for gargling, but for drinking, these oils must be removed. After three minutes the oils are boiled away and the vital enzymes are released which are important for the health of all glands, the bone marrow and the spinal discs.

Once the sage tea has been boiled, you should add one teaspoon each of St. John's wort (*Hypericum perforatum*), peppermint and balm (*Melissa officinalis*). Then let everything steep for another ten minutes.

Sage tea is the one I classify as the most important of all the teas. It should be drunk throughout your life. It was not just idle talk when a Roman scientist said: "Why die when sage can be grown in your garden?" He meant, of course, "Why die prematurely?"

2. Kidney Tea

My mixture:

> 15 g (0.53 oz) horsetail (*Equisetum arvense*)
> 10 g (0.35 oz) stinging nettle (*Urtica dioica*) (Nettle is best collected in springtime)
> 8 g (0.28 oz) knotgrass (*Polygonum aviculare*) (also called bird grass)
> 6 g (0.21 oz) St. John's wort (*Hypericum perforatum*)

This quantity will last one person for approximately three weeks. Place a pinch* into one half cup of hot water, let steep for 10 minutes, then strain out the tea leaves and set aside the liquid. Add another cup of hot water to the strained tea leaves, then boil for 10 minutes. After this, strain and pour the two liquids together.

*A pinch: the amount you can hold between your thumb and two fingers, for coarsely cut herb; if finely cut, take half a tablespoon.

Many people ask why kidney tea is prepared like this. Kidney tea contains five substances which must not be boiled away. But there is a sixth substance, silica (silicic acid), which dissolves only after 10 minutes of constant boiling.

Kidney tea treatment is to be taken for only three weeks. One quarter cup (60ml), taken cold, should be sipped on an empty stomach first thing in the morning; take another quarter cup just before lunch and the last quarter cup at night before going to sleep. During this time all meat should be avoided.

Kidney tea should be taken during every illness for a period of three weeks. It is especially important before surgery and when suffering from infections and inflammations. As a disease preventative, the kidney tea treatment can be taken three or four times a year, but allow intervals of at least two to three weeks between treatments.

3. Cranesbill Tea

Steep a pinch of leaves of herb Robert (Geranium robertianum, also known as red cranesbill) in one half cup of hot water for ten minutes. Slowly sip one half cupful of cold tea each day. If you notice any side effects, consult your naturopathic physician.

Cranesbill tea is vital for all malignancies, especially if you have received radiation treatment, because the tea contains a small amount of radium.

Notes on the Total Cancer Treatment

I am often asked questions. For instance, "Can I eat a little bread, honey, eggs or vegetables during the cancer treatment?" "Can I drink black currant, raspberry or pumpkin juice during the treatment?" People also ask whether they can take medicines during the treatment.

In The Correct Way to Follow My Treatment, in Part II, the Total Cancer Treatment is described in detail and it is to be followed exactly as I have prescribed. The juices are to be taken as indicated. A little lemon juice can be added but never apple juice! Freshly squeezed apple juice is allowed in between by itself but never mixed with the other juices. You may drink as much sage tea with St. John's wort, peppermint and balm as you want, but do not add any sugar.

It is preferable not to eat anything. By not taking notice of what I have said, i.e. by taking additional food or medicines (with the possible exception of insulin for diabetes – in which case consult your physician first), the result would take much longer or the treatment course may not work at all. In my personal opinion, if you do not rely solely upon the mentioned vegetable juices and teas, my treatment will not work! Over the years I have noticed that so-called failures of the treatment could be attributed to patients not following it in all aspects.

An estimated 40,000 cancer patients and others suffering from seemingly incurable illnesses have regained their health through my juice treatment. If patients are given medications which destroy cancer cells, the healthy cells will unfortunately be destroyed as well. In my opinion, cancer cells are not ill body cells, but just autonomous cancer cells. These cells can live only from substances contained in the foods we eat but they are not able to live on vegetable juices.

A cancerous tumor is an independent growth which produces independent cells. In a way, it cannot be classed as a disease. Naturally, this tumor presses on the endogenous cells and disturbs them, which is the actual illness. Therefore, we must destroy the cancerous cells by starving them with the juice fast. That is my opinion which I have gained from experience and I can prove it a thousand times over.

In Can Cancer be Healed?, in Part II, I described what a cancerous tumor is. Why such a tumor grows so slowly in the beginning and, in the final stages, grows so quickly, can be explained as follows:

One cancerous cell will double by splitting into two, then four, then eight, then 16 cells. That means that by the time 10,000 cells become 20,000 the continuous enlargement of the cancerous tumor proceeds very fast. But remember, the patient has still got the chance to be healed by the Total Cancer Treatment.

I would now like to implore all medical doctors and scientists to scientifically test my success in treating cancer and other seemingly fatal diseases, helping me help these suffering people rather than working against me just because I am not a medical doctor.

Just think about how many things have been done by people who do not have the legal qualifications. In the final analysis, the main thing is to help the people who are suffering in any way possible.

I beg you to remember how many great inventions were made by lay people. The most important thing, in the end, is the success of an idea and its usefulness for mankind. Scientists should acknowledge this fact, even if they cannot yet explain it. They should not care with whom or where the invention originated.

It often happens in science that something is being researched and that 60-odd years later the research goal still has not been reached. Now imagine that at that point an ordinary man, simple but gifted, finds the right answer, "maybe" accidentally, and achieves something, such as the successful treatment of cancer patients. I ask you, how can science and orthodox medicine simply ignore these successes and even refuse to test the applied method? I would therefore ask once again, that the ladies and gentlemen who are trained in medicine acknowledge the medical and technical successes of my method, even if there are certain aspects which they do not understand.

I would be extremely happy if you could improve my Total Cancer Treatment even more by combining it with other successful methods of cancer therapy.

Other Observations Regarding My Vegetable Juice Treatment

It is good to have a lot of exercise and fresh air!

I would like to point out that while my juice treatment has helped many cancer patients, it is also recommended for the following:

1. As prevention of cancer.
2. As a regeneration treatment for the whole body. Take 1/8 to 1/4 liter (1/2 to 1 cup) per day. Before eating always drink a small amount of the juice and the teas (sage tea and kidney tea).
3. For slimming without suffering from hunger and thirst and without damage to the body. If possible, continue the treatment for 42 days as recommended for the cancer treatment.
4. As a spring time elimination treatment.
5. To cleanse and improve your blood.
6. For joint illnesses, such as arthritis, in conjunction with the water treatments described in Part III.

Cancer patients who do not give up smoking for good will not benefit from my juice treatment at all!

If the cancer is far advanced, it is probably better if you can make the juice yourself from organically grown vegetables. Make sure to follow the juice mixture recipe precisely.

However, I am happy that a company is now manufacturing my "Breuss Vegetable Juice." I refer you to the suppliers under Resources at the end of this book. They guarantee that the mixtures are made from organically grown vegetables, as there are many thousands of people who do not have the time to make these juices fresh every day or are not able to obtain fresh, organic vegetables.

My Vegetable Juice Also Helps for the Following Illnesses:

Arthritis, arthrosis (degenerative joint inflammation), coxarthritis (hip joint arthritis), osteoporosis (bone decalcification), spondylarthrosis (arthrosis of the dorsal and lumbar vertebrae). For all these conditions the juice treatment has to be taken for only three weeks. Except for length of time, instructions are exactly the same as for cancer treatment, including taking the kidney and sage teas. (Should you want to do the treatment for the full 42 days, it certainly will not harm you. On the contrary, you would be sure that the body is now free of any cancer cells that might have been present).

With all the diseases of the joints, every third or fourth day a full bath is recommended to which horsetail (*Equisetum arvense*), hay flowers (*Graminus flos*), (also called grass flowers) or oat straw are added. Also recommended is the bath product "Herb-aku-cid" ("Kombi-Galvan-Badezusatz" from J. and S. Haubenshmid, Institut für Physikalische Therapie, Quellenstr. 21, CH-8580 Amriswil.) This product has been tested by the above Institute.

Important Supplementary Comments According To My Latest Findings

June 1987

This is written as a consolation for people living with cancer.

Cancer is not really a disease. It is just an independent growth which can develop - especially if one sleeps over water veins - and which can live only on solid food taken into the body. This is my conviction.

• With my Total Cancer Treatment such a growth is simply starved off. The juice mix and the teas contain all minerals, vitamins and trace elements the body needs during these 42 days.

• Since cancer is not a disease but simply an independent growth, medication does not really help, not even homeopathic or other natural remedies! Such a growth, then, can only be starved off with the juice treatment - as already described.

• According to my latest findings one may, or even should, take one to two bowls of onion broth a day (Caution: Take only the liquid, not the onion). I have given this broth to those who could not make it through the usual treatment because they were too weak. After adding it, everything went well. If, however, there is no need for this broth, it can be omitted, or one bowl could be eaten at noon only. (If you have only one bowl, never take it at night).

• Since it seems advantageous to the healing process, I can wholeheartedly recommend this onion broth to all cancer patients. With this broth they suffer from neither hunger nor thirst during the Total Cancer Treatment. There will be no complications and even those are helped who have had radiation treatments or chemotherapy.

• To support the heart, 20 to 40 drops of hawthorn tincture (*Crataegus oxyacantha*) should be taken in the morning, according to body size.

• Patients with cancer who also suffer from diabetes should continue insulin treatment during the juice fast. Besides that, any other medication will render my Total Cancer Treatment useless.

• **Caution**: With liver or gall bladder cancer never eat a whole bowl of onion broth in one sitting. It is best to take around 10 tablespoons of the warm liquid every hour. In addition, drink 1/2 cup (125 ml) wormwood (*Artemisia absinthium*) tea per day. Preparation of wormwood tea: The first five or six days steep one small pinch of wormwood in hot water for 10 seconds. After that, steep for only three seconds because otherwise it will be too strong!

Preparation of Onion Broth

Cut an onion, the size of a lemon, into small pieces without removing the outer brown skin. Roast the onion golden brown in a little olive oil, then add 1/2 liter (2 cups/500 ml) cold water. Cook until onion is soft, then stir in a vegetable bouillon cube. Pass the broth through a sieve taking only the clear liquid, without the onion.

You will find this broth very tasty.

The Correct Way to Follow My Treatment

Those who follow the Total Cancer Treatment (vegetable juice and tea) correctly will not lose much weight.

First thing in the morning, slowly drink a quarter cup (60 ml) of cold kidney tea. Thirty to 60 minutes thereafter sip one half to one cup of warm sage (*Salvia officinalis*) tea with St. John's wort (*Hypericum perforatum*), peppermint (*Mentha piperita*), and balm (*Melissa officinalis*). After an additional 30 to 60 minutes take a small mouthful of the juice mixture. Do not swallow it right away but allow it to get thoroughly mixed with saliva in your mouth. After approximately 15 to 30 minutes take another small mouthful of vegetable juice or wait until hungry again. During the morning take the juice approximately 10 to 15 times but only if you crave it. In between drink sage tea, which can now be taken cold and in any desired quantity. However, never add sugar during the juice treatment.

At noon drink another quarter cup (60 ml) of kidney tea and so again in the evening before going to sleep. Remember to drink the kidney tea only during the first three treatment weeks! In the afternoon the patient will frequently need a mouthful of the juice. No more than one half liter (2 cups/500 ml) of juice per day is allowed, but less may be taken.

When following my Total Cancer Treatment (6 weeks) and the Half Treatment (3 weeks), I must caution that the vegetable juice made as I describe must be taken as specified and in conjunction with the teas. Do not drink the vegetable juice alone! Take it only by the mouthful and mix with saliva.

Another important factor (whether or not the patient has received radiation treatment) is to take one half cup of cold cranesbill tea (herb Robert, *Geranium robertianum*) per day, sipping it by the mouthful. As mentioned before, cranesbill tea contains a small amount of radium. Remember the importance of slowly sipping your liquids which, by necessity, mixes them with saliva thus aiding your digestive tract.

During the treatment it is best to do a little work to take the mind off both eating and illness rather than rest in bed most of the time!

Besides the kidney tea and sage tea, some special cases (cancer in different areas of the body) require additional teas, as follows:

For Constipation:
If the constipation becomes bothersome, it is a good idea to start a series of enemas using camomile tea (*Anthemis nobilis*), or to drink a mild laxative tea or to gently insert a piece of hard butter into the anus.

Because of the juice treatment, the blood in the portal vein becomes so stimulated that whatever is in the intestines is fully utilized by the body. Therefore it can happen that over a period of a few days the patient has hardly any bowel movements or even none at all, but suffers no discomfort.

Cerebral Tumor:
One half to one cup of balm mint (*Melissa officinalis*) tea per day. Swallow it slowly when cold. Place a pinch of gold balm mint, lemon balm mint or mixed leaves in one half cup of hot water and let steep for 10 minutes.

Cancer of the Eyes:
One half cup of cold eyebright tea (*Euphrasia officinalis*) per day, also swallowed slowly. Steep a pinch of the herb in one half cup of hot water for 10 minutes, strain and let cool.

Breast, Ovarian and Uterine Cancers:
Drink one half cup of cold silvery lady's mantle (*Alchemilla alpina*) tea and white dead nettle, also known as blind nettle (*Lamium album*). Swallow slowly. To prepare, take a pinch of silvery lady's mantle tea, add a small pinch of white dead nettle (*Lamium album*) and steep in one half cup of hot water for ten minutes.

Cancer of the Gums, Lips, Tongue, Neck Glands and Larynx:
Use pimpernel tea (*Pimpinella magna*) as in diphtheria (see Alphabetical Listing of Illnesses, in Part III) but drink throughout the entire 42-day treatment. Put a tablespoonful of this tea into your mouth, rinse your mouth with it or gargle and then spit it out again. Do the same with the second tablespoonful. With the third tablespoonful do the same, but this time swallow. Do this several times per day. To prepare, put one teaspoonful of pimpernel herb into one half cup of water and boil for three minutes.

Skin Cancer (approximately ½ to 1 cm in diameter):
Swab the affected parts several times daily with fresh greater celandine juice (*Chelidonium majus*). The herb yields a yellow, bitter juice when plucked. If the spot is quite large, swab **only around** the part touching the healthy skin. In winter use greater celandine herb tea for swabbing or washing, but only around the affected area. Put a pinch of greater celandine herb into one half cup of hot water and let steep for 10 minutes. Apply still lukewarm. I must caution you again not to apply this solution to open wounds!

Bone and Lung Cancer and Lung Tuberculosis:
Drink tea made from plantain lance (*Plantago lanceolata*) or broad-leaved plantain (*Plantago major*), Iceland moss (*Cetraria islandica*), lungwort (*Pulmonaria officinalis*), ground ivy (*Glechoma hederacea*), mullein (*Verbascum thapsus*) and Meum mutellina herb. These teas are rich in calcium. Put the herbs together in hot water and steep for 10 minutes. (Not all these herbs need to be included in the tea). You can drink as much of this tea as you want, the more the better. To treat tuberculosis I recommend swallowing one teaspoonful of broad plantain lance per day with some water or tea.

Cancer of the Liver:
Drink one hot or cold cup of potato peeling tea per day. Put a handful of raw potato peelings in one cup of hot water and boil for two to four minutes. If this tea tastes agreeable, then the liver needs it! If it tastes disagreeable, you do not need it!

If you suffer from cancer of the liver, prepare cabbage packs or compresses, then rub the affected areas with olive oil or oil of

St. John's wort (St. John's wort steeped in olive oil). These cabbage packs or compresses are to be recommended to treat all forms of cancer and are best applied to the small of the back.

How to apply a cabbage pack:

Take three savoy cabbage leaves and wash them in warm water until there is no dirt left on the leaves. (The outside leaves are the best). Then roll the leaves with a bottle or rolling pin until all the veins on the cabbage are rolled flat.

To apply the pack put a folded wool blanket (folded approximately 50 cm/20 inches wide) on your bed. Place a linen cloth over top (approximately 25 to 30 cm/10 to 12 inches wide). On top of this place another cloth with the three cabbage leaves – (two leaves next to each other and one on top of them). Put the inside sheet with the cabbage leaves on the patient's back or onto the affected area, then wrap the linen cloth tightly over it with the wool cover on top. Fasten the pack as tightly as possible so it will not slip. (If it has not been applied properly and does not sit firmly in place, the patient will feel cold and could even start shivering, which would be very detrimental. If this happens, immediately remove the cabbage pack or compress.) The following morning take off the pack, wash the area with warm water and dry off thoroughly with a towel. Now rub one to two teaspoons of warmed oil of St. John's wort onto the affected area and put a warm towel over it. The towel can be removed a few minutes later.

Before you undertake the cabbage leaf wrapping, the patient must be covered warmly. It is best for the patient to be already resting in a bed that has been pre-warmed with a hot water bottle.

The booklet *The Fabulous Healing Power of the Savoy Cabbage Leaf* is available only in the French and/or German language edition and can be obtained from: Camille Droz, Herbalist, CH 2206 Les Geneveys-sur-Coffrane NE, Switzerland.

Cancer of the stomach:

One cup of wormwood tea or lesser centaury tea swallowed daily and cold. A small pinch for only three seconds in a cup of hot water to draw. Should your stomach still feel jumpy, then also drink a cup of valerian tea with wormwood every day: 1/2 teaspoon of valerian root in a cup of water and cook for three minutes, then in three seconds pour over a small pinch of wormwood.

Spleen and Pancreatic Cancer:

Drink at least one liter of warm or cold sage tea per day. Also recommended is a hot wrap made from hay, horsetail (*Equisetum arvense*) or oat straw. The hay flowers are left to steep, horsetail and oatstraw are boiled for 10 minutes (Only prepare this wrap if you know how to do wraps. You can do more damage than good if this procedure is not followed correctly). Instructions for this can be found in books on Kneipp therapy.

Prostate and Testicular Cancer:

Daily sip one cup of cold tea made from the small-flowering willow herb (*Epilobium*). Put a pinch into hot water and steep for 10 minutes.

All Cancers:

I have noticed that a tea rich in calcium such as the ones I recommend for use with bone and lung cancer is also good for patients with other types of cancer I can highly recommend this tea. The patient will not experience any lack of calcium or potassium while drinking this tea for treatment.

Completion of The Total Cancer Treatment

As I have said earlier, I always suggested medical supervision during the Total Cancer Treatment. I have done that so that the doctors could observe with me the progress of the treatment and the patient's health. They could check the patient's blood pressure and if the blood pressure was too low, prescribe a heart medication.

However, over time I have found that many orthodox medical doctors do not believe in this type of natural healing or natural remedies and will try to talk their patients out of taking this juice treatment. During my treatment the patients must not receive radiation treatment or injections. I know that it is not correct to proceed with my treatment without consulting the attending physician, as there could be complications. I must leave it to each individual to decide whether or not they request the supervision of their medical doctor. To check your own blood pressure, please refer to the Alphabetical Listing of Illnesses, in Part III, under "Blood Pressure."

Immediately following an operation patients must not start the Total Cancer Treatment. Wait at least two to five months, depending on how the patient feels. During the waiting period the patient should drink about 60 to 125 ml (a 1/4 to a 1/2 a cup) of vegetable juice per day, but he should also eat food such as gruel soup, vegetable soup, vegetables and maybe chicken or veal or other light foods. Before each meal, sip the juice and drink the teas I have recommended earlier, i.e. sage tea and kidney tea as suggested in the Total Cancer Treatment. Only start the Total Cancer Treatment when you feel well and strong enough.

Following the 42-day vegetable juice treatment, slowly start to eat light food again. It is very important that the food is salt reduced. Read nutrition books and favor light foods. Simultaneously, for a further two to four week period, continue to take approximately 60 ml (or a quarter cup) of vegetable juice per day. Take one mouthful at a time prior to eating your meals. To feel better much faster, three times daily take a teaspoon of Bio-Strath Elixir, or two Bio-Strath Yeast Tablets.

These natural remedies can be taken for a few months or until you feel well again.

I would like to mention that older people have an easier time with my cancer treatment. The older body does not require that many building materials, so fasting is not too hard.

Of about 40,000 successful cases I have personally treated more than 2,000, and I have said to each patient, "If you have any other acquaintances or relatives who also suffer from cancer, please tell them about my juice diet. Tell them to pass it on to others as well."A man once told me that he had followed my juice treatment exactly as I recommended. After just one week he noticed that he felt much better. He then recommended this treatment to another seven cancer patients and all of them recovered. I have asked my patients to pass on the details of the treatment because people kept coming from far away (from Hamburg, Lübeck and all parts of Germany, from Holland, Belgium, Switzerland, Canada, USA, etc.). I told these people to think of others who were not able to travel this far. By passing on the treatment from person to person, many patients with cancer and other seemingly incurable diseases can be helped.

In 1950 I healed my first cancer patient with the Total Cancer Treatment. I have now successfully treated cancer of the breast, brain tumors, cancer of the throat, cancer of the glands, lung cancer, cancer of the liver, bone cancer, intestinal cancer, etc. I have also healed those who had received radiation treatment and had badly burned skin because of it. You don't need to be so frightened of cancer any more!

Most cancer patients and seemingly terminal patients sleep above damaging water veins. (See the end of Part III.) In bad cases they lie on water veins which cross each other. The safest thing to do is to get a dowser to visit. He can tell where your water veins are. Then move your bed or sleep in another bed in a clear location.

[Editorial comment: Readers wishing to find out more about Ground Radiation and Earth Currents might wish to read the book: *Earth Currents – Causative Factor of Cancer and Other Diseases* by Gustav Freiherr von Pohl – Frech Verlag.]

PART III

Treating Leukemia and Other Illnesses

On October 1, 1952, I discovered that leukemia is not cancer of the blood but a decomposition of the blood because the portal vein circulation is diseased. This disease responds to treatment in most cases and with it the so-called leukemia.

On October 1, 1952, I was taken to see a lady (Regina Lorünser), who suffered from leukemia. Before I went into the lady's sick room, her husband, Robert, told me that she suffered from leukemia and had been to various medical doctors from Feldkirch to Dalaas. All of them had come to the conclusion that she had leukemia.

I asked him why he had asked me to come, because even I knew that leukemia could not be treated. He replied, "She doesn't know what her ailment is and we want to fulfill her every wish until her death. Because she heard about you and wanted to see you, why not try to cheer her up a little and comfort her?" I replied, "You mean more or less lie to her."

I then went to the lady and made an iris diagnosis of the eye for my own information simply because there is no book that tells you how to diagnose leukemia by studying the iris. If so many medical doctors have come to the conclusion that she suffers from leukemia, I thought to myself, then it must be correct.

During the diagnosis I could see that leukemia was not cancer of the blood but rather, a decomposition of the blood caused by the diseased portal vein circulation. This disease, in turn, is caused by mental depression, as was the case here.

Once I had made my diagnosis, I knew immediately how to treat her. I then told her what I was going to do and started with a quick compress as she had a fever of 40 degrees centigrade (104° F). As I was leaving, her husband said to me, "You have now told my wife so much that she believes she will get better."

I replied, "I know she will get better."

He didn't believe me and replied, "I have already told you that many doctors have said the same thing and what about the medical report from the [university] clinic?"

I said, "I don't care if a hundred doctors have told you that she is going to die. I tell you that she will recover."

"But Breuss," he said, doubtfully. I said to him, "I know exactly what you are thinking. You think that I am conceited or maybe even a fool. But, my dear Robert, by diagnosing your wife's eyes I have just discovered what exactly leukemia is. Therefore it is not dangerous anymore and all I can say to you is to follow everything exactly as I would in your place."

Mr. Lörünser then said, "Come here and look in the encyclopedia. There it says that to this day no one has been cured of leukemia."

I replied, "Then there were even more than 100 medical doctors involved," and added again, "Your wife will get well. Just carry out my instructions as I would carry them out myself." I then drove home and became inquisitive. That evening I read through my encyclopedia.

After reading the definition of leukemia, I was not so sure of my decision. One week passed by and I could not bear it any longer. So I got on my bicycle and went to visit the lady. When I arrived, I saw her working and she told me that on the fourth day she was already in the kitchen to help a little. This lady died five years later in a car accident! In 1978, in the space of ten months, 28 leukemia patients came to me and they could all work after six days. It is a portal vein circulation disease, not cancer of the blood. So far 150 leukemia patients have come to me and I could help all of them. Do not fear this disease any more.

What Do You Do When You Have Leukemia?

First of all, you have to decide what frame of mind you are in. As I have mentioned before, the functions of the portal vein circulation are damaged because of depression. This depression can often be caused by a simple thing. Often the patient himself does not know why he is depressed. Therefore, dear leukemia patients, try to find out the cause of your depression and then try to eliminate it through deep relaxation. Once you have done that, you have already achieved a lot.

For the treatment: Each day drink ¼ liter (1 cup) vegetable juice from the mixture of the Total Cancer Treatment but do not do the complete treatment.

Aside from drinking the juice you can eat what you enjoy except no beef soup and no pork. (Ed. note: Avoid any chemical food additives or burnt food and fats.) Drink the vegetable juice by swallowing it slowly. Use it throughout the day but especially shortly before meals.

The portal vein circulation system collects the concentrated vitamins, whether or not it wants to. It is also important to take careful note of the information on kidney tea, sage tea, as well as the warnings about warmed-up meals and poisons throughout the text. Everyone who does this treatment, should be able to work again as before, after approximately six days, even if the medical doctors say that he does not have much chance of survival.

It is most important that you drink ¼ liter (1 cup/8 fl oz) of juice per day for at least 42 days. Should you suffer from any other illnesses, these should be treated at the same time, as outlined on the appropriate pages of this book. Almost impossible to heal are those patients who are depressed and cannot overcome severe inner conflicts. You should also make sure that you have no moth powder, insecticides, sprays or air fresheners in the house. This is very important.

Why Illnesses Often Cannot Be Healed in Spite of Correct Diagnosis and Treatment

On April 24, 1944, I bought a book on diagnosing the iris of the eyes, *Der Krankheitsbefund (Diagnose) aus der Regenbogenhaut der Augen*, published by Dr. Otto Wirz (Württemberg) K.-Rohm Verlag (unfortunately no longer available).

Reading this book, I discovered why patients could not recover for 10, 20, 30, 40 or more years, even when they were diagnosed correctly and received the correct treatment. Dr. Wirz says, among other things, that the sprays used to kill moths and cockroaches contain naphthalene and camphor which in turn contain arsenic. This has been analyzed. If breathed in, these vapors can cause all kinds of diseases. He continues to say, "This poison [arsenic] is the greatest murderer of mankind. Its symptoms never disappear completely from the iris, which is a sign that this poisoning is more or less incurable."

Drawing from my many years of experience I could go into much more detail but I am convinced that one cannot heal a disease in a home where these poisons: naphthalene, camphor, DDT, fly spray, air cleaner, etc. are kept.

A Few Examples from Thousands of Cases

In 1944, the wife of a lawyer (Alice B.) came to see me and asked me to examine her. By diagnosing the iris of her eyes I came to the conclusion that she suffered from a serious skin disease. She agreed and informed me that was why she had come to me as she had suffered from this disease for 42 years. By this time she had consulted numerous physicians and dermatologists. There had never been a single moment of improvement.

I examined her more thoroughly and discovered that she suffered from an unusual poisoning caused by naphthalene. Breathing in these poisonous gases made it impossible for her to recover, even with the best treatment.

The woman doubted my diagnosis and stated that she had absolutely no naphthalene in her home. I replied, "I bet you 300

Marks that you have naphthalene in your home." She said that I would lose this bet. I replied, "Not I, but you are the one who will lose." She then said that she lived alone in her home, her husband had died and all her children were married. She should know if she had naphthalene in her home or not. I replied, "I know I'm right anyway, because it shows up so clearly in your eyes – like a photograph."

I then wanted to give her a tea for drinking, and another one for washing her diseased skin. But she wouldn't accept the tea, said I could drink it myself and remarked to the woman who had accompanied her, "Come on, let's go, once again I have wasted my time." Just before she left, I told her that I would go to her house the next day and then she would see that I would find naphthalene in her home. She replied, "You have no need to come as it will be a wasted trip."

Early the next day I did go to call on her. When she opened the door and I greeted her in a friendly manner, she immediately said, "So, you have come even though I have told you there is no point."

I then replied, "It doesn't matter. I have come to visit you for two reasons."

"What do you mean?" she asked.

"First, I have come to help you. Second, I would like to confirm whether my diagnosis is correct or not, so please let me in, because I mean well."

I was barely past the front door when I turned to the woman and asked whether she would like to increase the bet to 1,000 Marks. She looked at me stunned. Then I told her that the bet was not really fair, because I could already smell the naphthalene, which I quickly found.

She had a large wrought-iron candlestick with a candle approximately the size of a liter bottle. It was a fake candle used for show – and it was made from naphthalene.

49

"Now what do you say to that?" She said that she had lost the bet and became very friendly.

She then explained that she had been given the candlestick as a present years ago. It came from England. When she first received it, it was over one metre tall and approximately 10 to 15 cm in diameter. She was given the candle with the remark that it would be a nice decoration for her front room and that she would never have to bother about moths or cockroaches after that. Her home smelled like a poison chamber of naphthalene.

She then removed the candle and burned fragrant resin (German "Duftharz") in her home (You could also use holy incense). Thereafter she accepted my advice, drank the tea and washed the diseased areas with the other tea. Fourteen days later her skin disease was healed.

My dear readers, is this not sufficient proof that in a house containing this poison (arsenic) nothing will help the patient until the poison is removed and the home cleared with incense?

Another example: In May 1965 I was visiting the sanitarium "Maria vom Sieg" in Wigratzbad. There a woman approached me and asked if I could help. Her twelve-year-old daughter had become blind. The ophthalmologist had informed her that the cause was paralysis of the optic nerve and that no operation or glasses would help. As she had not brought her daughter along, I examined the iris of the mother's eyes and diagnosed that she must have a considerable amount of naphthalene in her house which was the reason why her daughter could not be helped. She told me that throughout the whole house every drawer contained this poison. I then told her mother exactly what to do and how to treat her daughter and that the girl would regain her sight within three weeks if she followed my instructions correctly.

Three weeks later, when I was in Wigratzbad again, this woman came to see me and informed me that her daughter could once again see normally and without glasses. You can imagine how glad I was! Just to witness the happiness in the mother's eyes was enough.

I then told the mother, "Take your daughter right away to see the ophthalmologist. Tell him without delay that your daughter would never have regained her sight if this poison had not been removed. Also inform him of my treatment so he can use it on other patients who suffer from a similar affliction."

A third and drastic case: A woman from Hamburg who lived for a time in Bludenz came to me with a serious skin disease and asked me to help her. She told me that for three years she had suffered from large blisters. As regular as clockwork the blisters would appear for five days on her right thigh, five days on her left thigh, five days from her abdomen to her neck, five days on her back and on the back of her arms then once again on her right thigh, and so on. She explained that for three days she would get only small pimples and on the fourth day these would turn into large water blisters (always about 80 or more). When they became full to the bursting point she simply had to squeeze them because the itching was beyond endurance. On the fifth day everything would heal, but the following day it would all begin again as described.

I then asked her why she had never gone to see a doctor. She explained to me that she came from Hamburg and only believed in homeopathy and naturopathy and would not go for any other treatment.

"But why not?" I asked her, trying to console her by adding," Our medical doctors are good, too."

She then told me that police constable Mähr had told her about my healing successes and had recommended me to her. That was why she was consulting me for my help. I then examined the iris of her eyes and diagnosed that her condition was caused by naphthalene poisoning.

When I told her the cause she said, with tears in her eyes, "Now I'll get better." I asked her why she was so sure that she would get better. She replied that when she was still living at home her father worked as a pharmacist in a homeopathic pharmacy and he often said that if he ever found naphthalene, fly spray, DDT or something similar for moths and cockroaches in the house, he would disown her, because he would consider that as deliberate murder.

She eventually got married and because a bomb dropped on their house one night, she and her husband lost everything they owned. She ultimately began to build up her life again, and so that the moths and cockroaches would not get at their clothes, she put naphthalene in the cupboards and forgot what her father had always said. After talking to me she removed all the poisons from their home and burned fragrant resin incense daily for two weeks. She drank kidney tea and washed the infected areas with another tea, as I had told her. After three weeks she was healthy again.

How to Treat Skin Ailments

As far as I know, there are more than 10,000 skin diseases and no physician in the world can know all of them. They are often incurable because nobody knows what skin disease the patient is suffering from.

Well, whether you know what skin condition it is or not, first drink kidney tea and sage tea. Drink the kidney tea and sage tea for the first three weeks; and then continue drinking sage tea for the rest of your life. If your blood pressure is high enough, take a teaspoon of brewer's yeast three times daily to cleanse your blood. Wash your skin with sage tea which you have left to steep for 10 minutes in hot water.

Even better to use are the sage stems, which have to be boiled for three minutes. The important thing is to always use four washcloths, that is, always make enough tea to wet four washcloths or other cloths. Then wash your skin with one cloth, turn it over and wash with the other side. Put the infected cloth aside, wash your hands with warm water and soap (because the hands become infected from the first wash), then take the second cloth and repeat. Wash your hands and repeat, etc. The first cloth is very infected from your first wash, the second a little less the third a little less again, while the fourth is hardly infected at all.

After washing for the fourth time, do not dry yourself. Put on clean underwear and clean nightclothes and change the bed linen. Horsetail can also be used for this method. Horsetail herbs (*Equistetum arvense)* should be boiled for 10 to 15 minutes. It is often good to wash one day with horsetail and the next day with sage tea. You can do this cleansing twice daily, but then you have to put on clean underwear twice daily.

Four cloths are needed if you cleanse, for instance, one arm. If you suffer from skin disease on both arms, you will require eight cloths. Should various parts of your body be infected, still more cloths will be required. It can happen that a patient will need as many as 28 of them.

If you suffer from dandruff or any other scalp disease, get another person to pour a little tea on the scalp and wash it with his hands. A short time later repeat – maybe 10 times. Finally, dry off lightly. You can wash your scalp with warm or cold tea.

Moist dandruff can be eliminated surprisingly fast with a cabbage leaf pack. The savoy cabbage is the best to use. The cabbage leaves must be wrapped well, tightly and warm. If the leaves are not wrapped tightly to the body, the patient will feel uncomfortable! You must press the leaves with a bottle or rolling pin until the veins of the leaves are flattened. The cabbage leaves are twice as effective if you drink kidney tea at the same time.

There are many other diseases which can be healed with cabbage leaf packs. (See The Correct Way to Follow My Treatment, in Part II.)

A 23-year-old woman, for example, suffered from tuberculous pleurisy. She ran a fever of 41 degrees Celsius. The medical doctors had no hope of her recovering, so I advised that she apply a cabbage leaf pack which was to be left on over night. In the morning, the cabbage leaves were removed. They were black and slimy and smelled terrible. After she was washed with warm water, the cabbage treatment was renewed every twelve hours. As I had predicted, already after the first packs a rash appeared which was approximately 20 by 20 cm in size. On the fourth day her mother asked whether the treatment could be stopped because of the fierce rash. I told her it would be wrong to stop now, because the illness would return, since the rash was the reaction to it. After three weeks her daughter's skin had cleared up and she was completely healed from her illness.

Are There Such People as Hypochondriacs?

In my opinion there are, but out of every hundred who are thought to imagine their illnesses, there is never more than one hypochondriac rather than a full fifty per cent as many people and even some doctors believe. If a patient is seriously ill but his suffering cannot be diagnosed, he often goes through a terrible time, as the following report of my own experiences will show:

For eight years I brought up everything that I ate or drank. Whenever I ate anything, I suffered with terrible pains, and when I didn't eat, I felt I was starving to death. I would be sick mainly around midnight. Eventually I was taken to the hospital. The head doctor, who gave me a fluoroscopic examination, informed me that I had many gall stones. I did not believe him and begged him to operate on my stomach instead of my gall bladder. But he thought that he was right and performed surgery on my gall bladder. He found that I did not have any stones but said that my gall bladder was twisted, so that he had to take it out.

After this operation, my condition became even worse. My stomach had grown shut because of a previous operation on my abdominal wall. Two years later I had surgery for cancer of the stomach. The attending radiologist had diagnosed this condition. Well, I did not have cancer of the stomach. As I mentioned before, my stomach had grown together from the previous surgery. The surgeon then examined my bowels. He still did not find anything unusual. Thereafter, I was declared a hypochondriac. Somehow the intestinal exploratory surgery caused a shift of the intestines, and two years later I had to undergo another operation to have part of a healthy colon removed.

After another two years I just could not stand it anymore. I once again went to the hospital. Meanwhile, eight years had gone by during which I was constantly in pain while still bringing up everything I ate. Now take note of what happened to me this time.

I had already been lying in the hospital for 14 days, suffering unendurable pain. As usual, at midnight, I vomited and in the morning my mouth and tongue were covered with blood. What I had brought up was as caustic as alcohol and it made me unable to speak. Every morning two assistant doctors would come by and would always greet me mockingly, "Good morning, naturopath. He helps all these other people but cannot heal himself."

I couldn't even answer them because the pain in my mouth was so intense, but because for once I did want to answer them, I did not eat anything all day. The next day the two medical doctors arrived with the same quip. This time I answered them, saying, "You talk like little kids who don't know what they are talking about."

One of the doctors replied, "What did you say?"

"You behave like two children."

The doctor said again, "What? You are repeating it?"

"Yes, I am! And I will a hundred times over! Look at the crucifix. Christ at the cross was told the same thing 1900 years ago and you are repeating it like copy-cats. What I am suffering from is so simple that you don't need to be a medical doctor or herbalist to be able to diagnose it. If nothing can be taken into the stomach, it simply means that the stomach has fused together and only surgery will help."

The doctors replied, "You haven't got any stomach left because it was surgically removed."

I replied, "That's only written down on paper."

"Patients are often led to believe certain things, but we have got your report," said the doctors.

"I can assure you that I still have my stomach exactly like you do. I know exactly what you think of me: that I am a hypochondriac. As one medical doctor has already suggested, I should try to imagine myself well instead of ill, so I would become well. I told that doctor: "Exactly the same thing could be said to someone who has had his hand amputated. He can tell himself a thousand times over that he still has his hand, but when he looks down at his arm, it's just not there.'" I then asked these two doctors if they knew what blood sedimentation a hypochondriac had, but I got no answer. Then I said, "0-3 because he is actually healthy. But I have 84, and now I would like to ask you why the sedimentation rate of the blood is tested, if nothing can be deduced from it?" I went on to explain to them how one treats hypochondriacs. That certainly surprised them! "No matter what," I said, "never make fun of them."

Towards the end of our conversation they were very friendly and even admitted that they had made a mistake. They added that they had learned a lot through this conversation. Later, they reported everything to the head doctor who had always been nice to me. He then did a fluoroscopic examination which showed that I still had my stomach. The result was surgery to remove my stomach, which was completely obstructed. Following the operation, nine medical doctors were sent to me during rounds and the head doctor exclaimed, "Mr. Breuss, what suffering you have been going through all these years and only you knew what was wrong with you." This confession made me very happy. That was in the year of 1956.

I have related my story only to alert medical doctors to the sufferings a patient has to go through when he is not diagnosed correctly – and when he is told that he is imagining his illness. Add to that the psychological hurt, when other people look at him in a funny way and also add to it the material damage he suffers, not to mention the unnecessary medical costs paid by his medical insurance.

All I can say to every physician is that he should think very carefully before suggesting that a patient is a hypochondriac. After all, the fate of a human being is at stake. Besides, being a hypochondriac also means that the person is ill. I hope that I have not embarrassed anyone by narrating my experience because anyone can make a mistake. No one on this earth is infallible and the things that are ordained to happen to us will happen to us anyway.

Alphabetical Listing of Illnesses

Abdominal Dropsy
See *Dropsy* below.

Adrenal Gland Disease and its Symptoms
If the suprarenal glands are not producing enough sex hormones, the person could develop a white spot on the throat (in the region of the larynx), often on the arms and, in serious cases, on the whole body. These patients are often very sad and lose interest in everything. In order to regain the proper functioning of the suprarenal glands, sip one half cup of cold cranesbill tea (herb Robert, *Geranium robertianum*) per day. A pinch of herb Robert should be allowed to steep in one half cup of hot water for ten minutes.

Cranesbill contains a small amount of radium. In one half cup of this tea there is exactly the quantity of radium that is required by the suprarenal glands. This tea can be drunk for one whole year.

In addition, you should also do breathing exercises (See *Breathing Exercises*)

Agoraphobia *(Fear of Open Spaces)*
See *Claustrophobia* .

Alcoholism
If there is a heavy drinker in the family who has often intended to give up drinking but who has never succeeded, there is almost certainly poison in the home (moth balls or the like). Where such poisons are kept, it becomes impossible to heal any illnesses, and alcoholism is definitely an illness. I would like to add: it is an illness of a weak will. In such cases, the smallest joy or anger becomes an excuse to drink. Therefore, all poisons should be removed and fragrant resin (or frankincense) should be burned.

Anemia

To counteract anemia, drink approximately one and a half cups of stinging nettle tea (*urtica dioica*) per day. It is to be slowly sipped hot or cold. Put one to three pinches of nettle into hot water and steep for 10 minutes. Patients suffering from anemia should also eat nettle spinach. Nettles contain much more iron than garden spinach. Patients who do not suffer from diabetes should take a small teaspoonful of bee honey once a day, dissolved in luke-warm milk, coffee or tea. In addition, drink 125 ml (1/2 cup) of red beet root juice per day. It would be even better to take 250 ml (1 cup) of the juice mixture described in the Total Cancer Treatment. If you want to, you can take more than the amount stated. A few tablespoonfuls should always be taken before meals.

In addition, one should do the breathing exercises (as described under *Breathing Exercises*). Through the long exhaling process the lungs are completely emptied of air, and when one deeply inhales again, fresh oxygen reaches even the furthest parts of the lungs.

Oxygen is carried by the red blood cells.

Here is a recipe to renew the blood corpuscles which is also recommended for anemia:

Put 81 dried pears into a light red wine. Use enough wine to cover the pears. Let stand for 10 days in a warm place (in sunshine, if possible) and then begin treatment as follows:

In the morning of the first day eat one pear. On the second day eat one pear in the morning for breakfast and one at lunch time. On the third day eat one pear in the morning, one at lunch and one in night. On the fourth day eat two pears in the morning, one at lunch and one in the evening. On the fifth day eat two pears in the morning, two at lunch time, and one in the evening. On the sixth day eat two pears three times. On the seventh day eat three pears in the morning and two at lunch and in the evening. On the eighth day eat three in the morning and at lunch and two in the evening. On the ninth day eat three pears morning, noon and night.

From the tenth day on, begin to eat one less pear every day. Therefore, on the tenth day you do as on the eighth day, on the eleventh day as on the seventh, the twelfth day as on the sixth etc. At the same time drink only the amount of wine which will allow for the remaining pears to stay covered by wine. Drink the wine starting at lunch, not in the morning.

Apoplexy
See *Bleeding of Any Kind*

Appetite (Loss of)
Loss of appetite could be caused by the body not needing any food for a period of time, for example if one does not feel well. This is often the case with children. In such cases it is wrong to eat for the sake of maintaining regularity or to force a child to eat. Appetite returns on its own accord when the body is ready again. If for eight days such a child or adult is given one half to one and a half cups of *Meum mutellina* tea, it restores their lost appetite. The world-famous healer, Father Kneipp, says: "If you are hungry, then eat. If you are thirsty, then drink." Therefore, if you have no appetite, do not eat. There are people whose portal vein circuit absorbs the food into the body completely and therefore they do not require much food. Mentally ill persons usually have something wrong with their portal vein's function and therefore may have an exaggerated appetite. The portal vein circulation's role is to absorb the food from the stomach and intestines into the body. It can be compared with the fine absorbing roots of a tree.

Arteriosclerosis
Slowly sip one half to one cup of cold yarrow tea (*Achillea millefolium*) (also called milfoil) per day. Put one or two pinches of yarrow into one half to one cup of hot water and steep for 10 minutes. In addition to this tea, take one teaspoonful of brewer's yeast three times per day.

Brewer's yeast is one of the best means for blood cleansing, as is garlic. These are good remedies for treating arteriosclerosis.

Please note: All these remedies against arteriosclerosis tend to reduce blood pressure. Take them only when your blood pressure is not too low. It is a good idea to have a blood pressure meter at home for this purpose. If not, find out your blood pressure from your physician.

Arthritis

Arthritis usually occurs where poison is kept in the home, i.e., moth powder, naphthalene, camphor etc. The first thing to do, therefore, is to remove these poisons. After that, the treatment is the same as for rheumatism. When your knees bother you, I recommend the following exercise: several times a day without bending your knees, step heavily on one foot and then change to the other.

Should you have arthritis in your wrist, keep a stiff wrist and punch as if to push the wrist up into the forearm. (This wrist exercise is analogous to the knee exercise). Do this exercise several times a day. I also advise you to do the three week vegetable juice treatment.

Arthrosis

This requires the same treatment as arthritis. Take one to two tablespoonful of dandelion juice (*Taraxacum officinale*) daily in warm water. This is a very effective additional therapy.

Asthma

If the liver and gall bladder are functioning properly, drink onion tea for three weeks. Boil two egg-sized onions in their skins, in one liter (4 cups) of water with 100 grams (3 1/2 ounces) of dried sugar cane juice or other unrefined sugar for 10 to 15 minutes. Sip this cold throughout the day.

Often during the day eat a little black radish in its skin. This can also be eaten as a salad but without salt. In addition, drink a quarter liter (1/2 cup) of warm milk, wine or cider with Cinquefoil (*Potentilla anserina*), also called goosegrass, crampweed or silverweed. The preparation for this is described under *Cramps*.

Bad Breath

Bad breath usually means that something is wrong with the stomach. In this case drink one half cup of wormwood tea (*Artemisia absinthium*) per day (cold) for three to five weeks. Steep a small pinch of wormwood for only three seconds in one half cup of hot water.

Bad breath can also be caused by abscesses, brittle teeth or cavities. In this case, visit your dentist! Decayed teeth should always be immediately attended to or taken out. I would never recommend treatment for decayed teeth.

Basedow's Disease (Goiter)

This illness is not, in principle, an illness of the thyroid gland. The enlargement of the thyroid gland and the protruding eyeballs result from the trigeminus hammer nerve. This hammer thumps at a great speed on the trigeminus hammer nerve, thus causing various glands to be disrupted, some of which eventually stop working. As a result, the thyroid gland takes over their work, and that is why it grows larger. Should a person suffering from Basedow's disease be away from home, say on a three-week holiday, and have new experiences and interests every day, then the enlargement of the thyroid gland will disappear. This is a sure sign that this is a nervous disease. If a patient is exposed to the same monotonous surroundings all the time, then he will have constant trouble with his trigeminus hammer nerve. If you operate on the Basedow goiter, the substitute for the other glands will have been removed. Such patients then are more or less always ill. Instead of surgery performed on them, these patients should receive similar treatment as those suffering from neurasthenia, circulatory disorders, etc. Most important are the breathing exercises. (See *Breathing Exercises*.) By no means should there be poisons in the home.

Bed-Wetting

For this complaint each day drink one half cup of yarrow tea (*Achillea millefolium*) which has been left to steep for ten minutes in half a cup of hot water. In this disease the sphincter muscle of the bladder is insensitive. Yarrow tea re-awakens that feeling. It is often helpful to wrap a towel around the stomach of the bed-wetter and then tie a large knot behind, so that the patient cannot sleep on his back. Water can only be passed unnoticed when the bed-wetter is lying on his back.

Belching

See *Stomach Disorder (Gastritis)*.

Bile, Insufficient Production

If the stool is light or nearly white in color, this is a sign that the liver is producing too little or hardly any bile.

In this case you should drink tea made from potato peelings for a few days. Boil a small handful of potato peelings in one cup of water for two to four minutes. Keep taking a mouthful of the cold tea throughout the day.

Bilious Colic

See *Kidney and Gall Bladder Attacks*.

Birthmarks

See *Warts and Birthmarks*.

Bleeding of Any Kind

Should you suffer from stomach hemorrhage, intestinal hemorrhage, nosebleeds, bleeding of the gums or cerebral hemorrhage, you should take three drops of tormentil (*Potentilla tormentilla*) tincture [in Britain this is also known as bloodroot – not to be confused with the North American bloodroot (*Sanguinaria canadensis*)] twice a day, undiluted, or sip a cup of cold tormentil tea per day. The preparation of tormentil tea and tincture is listed under *Dysentery* below.

When bleeding of the gums occurs, after each meal clean your teeth, especially after eating anything sweet, and then rinse with tormentil tea and also drink a little of the tea. After approximately two weeks, you can take tormentil drops instead of tea.

In case of cerebral hemorrhage, you should take a cup of masterwort tea (*Imperatoria ostruthium*) in addition to the tormentil drops or the tormentil tea. You should take a sip of masterwort tea every hour. To prepare the tea, boil a teaspoonful of masterwort roots for three minutes in a 1/4 liter (1 cup) of water. Instead of water, a 1/4 liter of wine could be used. In this case, too, a sip of cold liquid should be taken every hour. This remedy is most effective when taken on the first day of the apoplexy.

Blood Pressure, Too High

To treat high blood pressure drink one half to one cup of yarrow tea (*achillea millefolium*) per day. In addition, three times a day take one teaspoon of brewer's yeast.

Besides these, also do the breathing exercises (See *Breathing Exercises*). Garlic and mistletoe (*Viscum album*) also work against high blood pressure. Try to avoid coffee, alcohol (especially red wine), camomile tea, pork and celeriac.

Blood Pressure, Too Low

To counteract low blood pressure, eat a lot of celeriac salad and strawberries or strawberry jam. If the liver is not causing any trouble, coffee is appropriate, as well as a little red wine and onion tea. To prepare onion tea, take two egg-sized onions including the skins and place into one liter (4 cups) of water together with 100 grams (3 1/2 ounces) of dried sugar cane juice. Boil for 10 to 15 minutes, let stand and sip cold. Also, take 15 drops of Salus-Haus or Dr. Vogel hawthorn tincture (*Crataegus oxycantha*) three times per day before meals. If there is no lunula or half-moon to be seen on the thumb nail of the left hand, also take 20 drops of Salus-Haus valerian tincture three to four times a day between two p.m. and the evening.

As with high blood pressure, the breathing exercises are also a good treatment against low blood pressure (See *Breathing Exercises*). Do not do too much work. However, not doing anything at all would be worse. If you do not put any demands on your heart, you will make it weaker still.

One can tell the state of one's blood pressure by looking at the finger nails of the left hand. The heart, so it is said, is a large muscle which is made up of a major and four minor muscles. If the moon shape of your thumb can only just be seen or not seen at all, then your main heart muscle is too weak. If this is the case, you must take 30 to 40 drops of valerian tincture (depending on the size of the patient) three to four times between three p.m. and evening.

If there is a half moon on your thumb but none on the other four nails, then your minor heart muscles are weak. In this case, take 20 to 30 drops of hawthorn (*Crataegus oxyacantha*) tincture three times a day (normally before meals). Take only hawthorn drops, never valerian drops.

If there is no half moon on any of your nails, then you require both valerian and hawthorn drops. In this case, also add about one half cup of celeriac juice, taken throughout the morning, one mouthful at at time. All these are completely natural remedies.

As far as determining blood pressure is concerned: little or no showing of the half moons means that your heart muscles are weak; therefore, you have low blood pressure.

Breathing Exercises

Breathe in through the nose, then breathe out through the mouth with the following sounds:

E, A, O, U, AA [as in "Baa baa black sheep"] and SH. [German I, E, O, U, A and SCH]

The "SH" is voiced, that is, accompanied by a continuous humming sound. The same effect can be gained by humming M through the nose with the mouth closed. Breathe in for about seven seconds, then "sing" - that is, breathe out - for seven seconds.

Do these exercises for five to ten minutes each time, the more often per day the better.

The "E" is for the brain, the eyes and the ears; the "A" is for the throat; the "O" is for the heart; the "U" is for the abdomen. The

"AA" is for the extremities (hands and feet), especially with paralysis. The M/SH is for the whole body. In the brain, these breathing exercises have the effect of a complete body massage. Because the exhaling takes so long, the lungs are completely emptied and oxygen can reach even the smallest parts of the lungs. This is another beneficial effect of these breathing exercises.

Bronchitis

If your liver and gall bladder are in good order, then bronchitis can be quickly healed with onion tea. Boil two egg-sized onions with their skin for 10 to 15 minutes in one liter (4 cups) of water with 100 grams (3 1/2 ounces) of dried sugar cane juice or other unrefined sugar added. Take in sips when the tea is cold.

Besides this tea, teas containing calcium may be taken, such as ribwort or plantain (*Plantago lanceolata*), greater plantain (*Plantago major*), Iceland moss (*Cetraria islandica*), and *Meum mutellina*. Not everyone of these herbs has to be put in the tea. Let all the herbs used steep together in hot water for ten minutes.

Buzzing of the Ears (Tinnitus)

This is mainly caused by too much blood rushing to the eardrum or irritation of the auditory nerves. Another reason could be the hardening of the eardrum or deposits of hard ear wax. Buzzing of the ears can often be remedied by *water-treading* (See *Water Treatments*) and, particularly, by *cold foot packs* which are left on overnight. But as in the case of water-treading, foot packs should only be put on during the moon's waning phase. In the case of ear wax deposits, the patient should go to an ear specialist for removal. This will immediately alleviate the problem.

To apply a *foot pack*, take a pair of wet cotton socks, wring them out well and put them on your feet. The wet socks should reach above the ankle. Put a pair of thick woolen socks over them and then wrap each foot well with a warm woolen scarf. Finally, wrap the feet together in a warm, woolen blanket. In this manner, the blood will be drawn to the feet, and this will reduce the rush of blood to the ears.

Follow these instructions carefully. If foot packs are not done properly, the opposite effect will occur.

All Kneipp water treatments should start on the right-hand side. This means that you should take care of the right foot first and then do the left one. This is very important!

You can also apply a savoy cabbage pack around the calves and leave on overnight. You need one or two savoy cabbage leaves for each leg, depending on size. They must be wrapped up exceptionally tight and then kept warm.

To prepare the cabbage leaves, dip in cold or lukewarm water in order to remove any dirt. Spread them out on a cloth and roll them with a bottle or rolling pin until the ribs are flat and smooth. (The ribs are an important part of the leaves, so never cut them away. For instructions for cabbage pack preparations, see The Correct Way to Follow My Treatment, in Part II.)

Cancer of the Prostate

See *Prostate*

Cataracts

In cases of cataracts (as with all illnesses) the patient should drink kidney tea for a period of three weeks. Sage tea should always be taken. Never eat reheated food!!!

Poison must not be kept in the home.

To fight the cataract itself, drink as much apple peel tea as possible, but only after four p.m. This is the best tea for the nerves. As far as I know, this is an illness caused by the nerves. To prepare the tea, boil the peel for three to six minutes.

Chilblains

In case of chilblains boil around 15, 20 or even more mashed horse chestnuts in three to five liters (12 to 20 cups) of water for one hour. The affected part should be bathed in this warm mixture for half an hour. The same mixture may be reheated and re-used twice if there are not enough horse chestnuts. For lighter cases, three or four of these baths should be enough, but for long-standing cases up to 12 baths may be required.

Chills and Shivers

For chills, take several half liter (2 cups/500 ml) bottles with tight-fitting caps or corks. Fill bottles with hot water, put inside wool socks and place between the arms and the body. Do the same between the legs – that is between the thighs and lower legs. In addition you should use four bottles for the outside part of the legs (two to the left and two to the right) and another one for the soles of the feet. The chest should be covered with a heating pad. In this way, shivers are normally relieved within ten minutes.

[*Editorial:* A more modern method would be to rub your entire body with Olbas Oil (available in health food stores) and immediately thereafter take a hot shower, as hot as you can stand it, and then go to bed.]

Childlessness *(infertility)*

If a married couple has been childless for some years and really wants to have a baby, I suggest that both partners take a half cup of cold cranesbill tea (herb Robert, *Geranium Robertianum*) every day. The tea should be taken slowly, one mouthful at a time. Usually there are quick results. A few years ago, eight women who had been married from two to ten years consulted me about this problem, all within a month. They drank this tea regularly and each one of them became pregnant after about four to six weeks. All of them gave birth to exceptionally beautiful and healthy children, which, of course, made them extremely happy.

To prepare the tea, steep a pinch of herb Robert (*Geranium Robertianum , also known as red cranesbill*) in one half cup of hot water for ten minutes. If this does not help, then the case is more or less hopeless.

Circulatory Disorders

If suffering from circulatory disorder, you almost definitely suffer from cold feet. Therefore it is of prime importance to alleviate this problem. One very useful treatment is the alternating foot bath (see *Water Treatments*). Another excellent treatment is Father Kneipp's water treading (see *Water Treatments*).

Claustrophobia/Agoraphobia

Claustrophobia is a phobia of enclosed spaces; agoraphobia is the phobia of large open spaces. People suffering from these phobias (irrational fears) have a serious deficiency of phosphorus. In order to supply the body with the required phosphorus, eat plenty of celery root (celeriac) salad and a lot of strawberries and strawberry jam. Wild strawberries contain more phosphorus than the cultivated varieties. Celery root holds more phosphorus than any other plant. It is best eaten raw. Grate the roots, add vinegar and freshly-pressed flax oil as you would with other salads. Add a little unrefined sugar. Kneipp says: "If there is vinegar, there should be sugar as well."

If you do not like celeriac salad raw, you can boil the roots, but make sure to drink the celery water because this will contain the phosphorus after the cooking process.

If you have a major exam coming, start eating foods rich in phosphorus three weeks beforehand, and you will pass the exam easily. Children who eat a lot of strawberries learn easier!

Colic

See *Kidney and Gall Bladder Attacks*.

Constipation

Several times a day eat a forkful of raw (homemade) sauerkraut or Eden sauerkraut from your health food store. Immediately afterwards drink a sip of water. Also drink approximately half a liter (2 cups/500 ml) of sage tea per day. People who always drink sage tea never suffer from constipation. Do not eat white bread or chocolate.

Convulsions in Babies

When a child gets violent fits of crying and convulsions, give him or her half a cup of chickweed tea (*Stellaria media*). This is a weed which grows in clumps in gardens, rich potato fields and mainly in vineyards between the vines. This half cup of tea should be drunk at one sitting, warm or cold.

Steep one pinch of **fresh** herbs for 10 minutes in one cup (250 ml) of hot water. Dried chickweed is of no use! In winter, prepare one leaf of house leek (*Sempervivum tectorum*) in the same manner. A child who is suffering from this complaint in its advanced stages and drinks this tea, will be much improved after one to two hours.

Chickweed tea is also good for unclear skin of the face or body. In this case, however, the tea must be taken over a longer period of time. The tea is also very good for the heart. During winter, house leek might be available at garden centers.

Coughs

To soothe a cough, drink onion tea as used in bronchitis. (See *Bronchitis.*) Boil two egg-sized onions with their skins in one liter (4 cups) of water. Add 100 grams (3 1/2 ounces) of dried sugar cane juice or other unrefined sugar. Boil for 10 to 15 minutes. Sip when lukewarm or cold.

Cramps

Boil a pinch of cinquefoil (*Potentilla anserina*) (also called goose grass, crampweed, silverweed) in a quarter liter (1 cup/250 ml ~ 8 oz.) of milk, wine or cider. Put the herb in cold liquid. As soon as it starts boiling, remove from heat and strain before drinking.

This remedy should be taken warm in the morning. Cinquefoil is ineffective if boiled in water.

If women suffer from *menstrual cramps* they should take this tea one or two days before and also during menstruation. After the first use, there will already be some improvement; after the second, it will be even better and after the third, better still. After the fourth time, the cramps are as good as gone.

Crooked Fingers

There are quite a few people who cannot straighten their fingers any more. Most affected are the ring or middle fingers. The little fingers are rarely involved. This condition is caused by flat feet or fallen arches. If the fingers of the right hand are affected, the fallen arches are on the left side. If the fingers on the left hand are affected, the foot problem is on the right side.

This opposite or crosswise reaction shows that the tendons are involved. The tendons are attached to the front part of the ball of the foot, run along the foot, the heel, the calf and the hip, and cross over at the lower part of the back. They then run up to the arms and to the fingers. If somebody has flat feet, it causes the tendons to be too tight. As they cannot be stretched, they pull in the fingers, at best. At worst, flat feet can cause changes to the hip joints because, as I have already mentioned, the tendons run along the hips. If the hips become distorted, the fingers will not be affected.

Regardless of whether it is the fingers or the hips which are affected, the best remedy is to use arch supports. Do not wear house slippers without arch supports. Then, at least, the condition or ailment will not get worse. In many cases, arch supports bring about a considerable improvement.

Even many medical doctors may not know that these bent fingers and strained hip joints are caused by flat feet. For example, I knew a woman who suffered from a seriously strained hip joint. For over 15 years the doctors had been treating her for rheumatism. I assured her that this condition was caused by flat feet and advised her to have an x-ray on the opposite foot. The same day she consulted a radiologist and had an X-ray done on her foot. He showed her the x-ray and remarked that the strained hip joint was caused by this fallen arch. If this woman had consulted the radiologist 15 years sooner, she would have been prescribed arch supports and the strained hip joint would never have occurred. In short, if you experience tightening of your fingers or changes in your hip joints, make sure to have an X-ray taken to diagnose fallen arches. Wear your arch supports all the time, even if they hurt at first.

Depression

See *Neurosis - Mental Disorder – Depression.*

Diabetes

To treat this disease, I recommend the Kneipp Spa Therapy, consisting of diet and hydrotherapy.

All sweet food is strictly prohibited, as well as alcohol and caffeine. White bread and any other food containing white flour should be avoided. Also stay away from fatty meat and meat broth.

I particularly recommend a diet of quark cheese*, which should be eaten in the evening for an extended period of time. Eat your food slowly, chew it well, and get a lot of exercise in fresh air!

Herbal remedies: Drink tea made from bean pods, herb Bennet (*Geum urbanum*) blackberry leaves, blueberry leaves, and golden cinquefoil (*Potentilla reptans*). Steep these herbs together for 10 to 15 minutes in one to one and a half cups of hot water. The tea should be sipped cold during the day. Furthermore, take three tormentil tincture drops (*Potentilla tormentilla* or *Tormentilla erecta*) once or twice per day. A regular check-up is very important.

*Quark cheese is a soft cheese made with rennet from sweet milk or butter milk. It is available in health food stores.

Diarrhea

See under *Dysentery.*

Diphtheria

For diphtheria gargle with pimpernel (*Pimpinella magna*) tea and also drink a little of the tea. Gargle with a tablespoon of the tea, then spit it out. Do the same with a second spoonful. With the third spoonful, gargle and swallow. Repeat this action every 90 minutes. This treatment works so well that it rarely has to be repeated the next day. To prepare the tea, boil a teaspoon of pimpernel roots in 1/4 liter (1 cup/250 ml) of water for three minutes. In addition, the patient can drink a spoonful of warm lemon juice every ten to fifteen minutes.

Diptheria is actually very rare these days and can be prevented by inoculation.

Dropsy of the Heart and Abdominal Dropsy

In the case of dropsy of the heart, take a tablespoonful of pure water every two minutes. Every half hour drink a spoonful of kidney tea instead of water. (Large people should take a large tablespoonful, smaller persons, a smaller one). However, those who have had a heart attack should take a spoonful every three minutes.

Many people still believe that those suffering from this disease should not even take one eighth of a liter (1/2 cup) of liquid per day. I do not agree with this. Of course, it all depends on **how** it is taken. If the patient drinks a quarter liter (one cup) at a time, he might die on the spot because his heart would not be able to cope with it. It is even possible that as few as three to four spoonfuls would be too much! For this reason, it is very important to take only one spoonful every two to three minutes. Always take liquids by the spoonful and never drink from a glass because even a small quantity in a glass could be more than a spoonful.

Everyone's heart can cope with taking a tablespoonful of water every two to three minutes. By means of this water treatment, the uric acid in the legs, which may amount to twenty liters (80 cups), is diluted. As a result of this, the viscous uric acid can escape from the tissue, by evaporation. For dropsy of the heart, this treatment will take only two days. On the second day, the patient will smell very strongly of urine. The term "dropsy of the heart" would be better named "dropsy of the heart/uric acid condition" because in this condition the uric acid is extremely viscous and cannot be secreted through the skin any more. This is my conviction. During this water treatment you are allowed to eat, but never drink water during meals. Resume the water treatment ten minutes after finishing a meal.

When suffering from abdominal dropsy, take a small sip of water every five minutes. In this case, however, it takes much longer for any success to be noticed.

Instead of water you can now and again drink sage tea, peppermint tea or balm mint tea – but, please, only by the spoonful.

Duodenal Ulcers

See *Stomach Disorders*

Dysentery

To treat dysentery and diarrhea, take three drops of tormentil tincture (*Potentilla tormentilla*) per day or drink 1/2 cup of cold tormentil tea, one mouthful at a time. To prepare the tea, boil a teaspoonful of the roots in 1/4 liter (1 cup/250 ml) of water for three minutes. The drops should be taken undiluted. A healing effect is only achieved by taking three drops. Four drops is too many. In this way, dysentery is healed within 24 hours.

It is very rare that dysentery will still occur on the second day and that another three drops are required. Of course, it all depends on how these drops are prepared. If you have the opportunity to prepare them yourself, then do so. To make a good and effective tormentil tincture, the roots should be collected in autumn, dried for three days and cut into small pieces. Put, in a dark bottle with schnapps (or vodka); use a handful of roots to a half liter (2 cups/500 ml) of schnapps (grain spirit). Do not fill the bottle completely. Leave for a full three weeks in a warm place, then strain. Add more roots to this tincture and leave for another three weeks in the sun (or warm spot). This process can be repeated for a third time. In this way you will obtain a tincture which is three times the normal strength and therefore very effective.

Fainting

Fainting may have a number of causes, for example, a sudden loss of blood to the brain or too much blood entering the brain, caused by unexpected sensations and emotions such as terror, fear or joy. Other causes are great pain; the narcotic effects of gas or alcohol; vibrations of the brain caused by a blow or a fall on the head; loss of blood; hunger; or a general deterioration caused by growing anemia.

The patient does not always faint immediately. The most important warning signals are attacks of dizziness and vision and hearing disturbances. If the patient does faint, his breathing and heart activities are very low. The forehead and limbs feel cold and the forehead is usually covered with cold sweat.

Fainting can be a symptom of various illnesses and may be a small side effect of a much more serious condition. In people who are susceptible to fainting the pupils constantly change with the rhythm of the patient's breathing before and after the attack. Their pupils contract, and then, the very next moment, enlarge to double or even triple their previous size. In such cases, *Meum mutellina* tea helps wonderfully. Unfortunately, this tea is not available everywhere. If you cannot obtain it locally, check the listing under "Resource List."

I once was at a veterinarian's home on business and I noticed that his wife's pupils were constantly changing as she was speaking.

I said to her, "Either you have fainted recently or you are soon going to."

She answered, "I fainted six times during the last week."

So I gave her some *Meum mutellina* tea and observed that although the tea did not taste very pleasant it would certainly do her good because she was greatly in need of it. She actually liked it so much that she drank more than 10 liters (40 cups) per day for 10 days. In the afternoon of the tenth day, she suddenly could not stand the tea any longer (because she did not need it anymore). She said, "If a drunkard enjoys wine or spirits as much as I enjoyed that tea, then I can understand why he cannot stop drinking."

In 1943, this woman had to go for lung examinations regularly. However, after the tea treatment she only had to go once more because the symptoms of disease had disappeared. Today, in 1980, she has not had a single fainting spell and she has not been ill. This means that tea made from the herb Meum mutellina is not only good for preventing fainting spells, but is also the best tea for both lung disease and anemia. You can drink as much as you like of this tea. It should be allowed to steep for 10 minutes in hot water.

If fainting is caused by a rush of blood to the brain, then *Meum mutellina* tea is not recommended because it is a marked stimulant. If someone faints, loosen all tight-fitting articles of clothing such as collars and ties. If the patient looks very red in the face, he should be propped up in an upright position. If the patient vomits, his head should be turned to the side. To stimulate the breathing and heart, it is best to sprinkle the chest and whole body with fresh water. Substances such as Eau de Cologne or ether will also have a stimulating effect if briefly held in front of the patient's nostrils.

Gall Bladder

See *Bile, Insufficient Production*

Also see *Kidney and Gall Bladder Attacks*

Gastric Ulcers

See *Stomach Disorders*

Gastritis

Inflammation of the stomach. See *Stomach Disorders*

Goiter *(Exophthalmic Goiter)*

See *Basedow's Disease*

Goiter *(Struma)*

In the case of goiter, sip half a cup of angelica root tea (*Angelica archangelica*) per day. This tea should be taken cold, in slow sips. A teaspoonful of angelica root should be boiled for three minutes in one half cup of water. One half cup of angelica root tea contains exactly the amount of iodine which the thyroid gland requires per day.

Grippe

See *Influenza*

Hay Fever

In the case of hay fever, you should clean your nose thoroughly before going outdoors. Then dip a Q-tip in fresh-pressed flax oil and dab inside the nostrils. You should keep some Q-tips and oil with you at all times to repeat the procedure each time you have to wipe your nose. If the nostrils are covered with oil, the pollen will not be able to cause any more irritation.

Headaches

There are people who suffer from stomach diseases but who never have trouble with their stomachs. Instead, they have very bad headaches over the eyes and forehead. These headaches are symptoms of the stomach disease. Such people will soon be healed if they sip one half cup of cold wormwood tea (*Artemisia absinthium*) per day for three to five weeks. They should take the tea cold, sipping a small amount every hour.

To prepare the tea, let a small pinch of wormwood steep for three seconds in one half cup of hot water (See *Stomach Disorders*).

For headaches which occur on one side only (*migraine*), balm mint tea (*Melissa officinalis*) is very beneficial. One pinch of golden balm or lemon balm should be left to steep for 10 minutes in one half cup of hot water. The tea should be sipped cold.

People who have headaches at the back of the head usually have trouble with the intervertebral discs in the neck region. This can be remedied by manipulation of the neck region. Blood pressure which is too low could also be at the root of the problem (refer to *Blood Pressure, Too Low*).

A good treatment for all these headaches is primrose tea (*Primula officinalis*) with St. John's wort (*Hypericum perforatum*). Mix both together and let steep for ten minutes in a cup of hot water. Also, sipping half a cup of violet tea (*Viola odorata*) every day often brings speedy relief, especially for nervous headaches. This tea should also be left to steep for 10 minutes in half a cup of hot water.

Heart Muscle

See *Myocardial Damage.*

Hemorrhoids

For this condition do cold water enemas once or twice a day for eight days using 1/4 liter (1 cup) of cold water. Discharge the enema immediately with several interruptions. Afterwards, hemorrhoidal ointment such as witch hazel cream should be applied.

If blood is discharged, also take three undiluted tormentil tincture drops (*Potentilla tormentilla*), once or twice a day. These drops can also be taken with honey or other unrefined sugar. However, bleeding should always be checked out by a physician.

Hiccups

For this problem, take a teaspoonful of caraway seeds and swallow with some water without chewing them. After two hours at the most, the hiccups will have ceased completely.

On July 28, 1964, when I was at the sanitarium "Maria vom Sieg" in Wigratzbad, a clergyman with this illness came to me. I assured him that he would be completely healed after two hours at the most. This clergyman told me with great difficulty, for he could hardly speak having hiccups every few seconds from morning to night, that for months he had consulted one doctor after another but without success. Then I told him that Pope Pius XII had died of this disease and that I was sure that in his case the best doctors had been consulted. I reassured him of what I had said and gave him a teaspoonful of caraway seeds. You will hardly believe this. After five minutes, he stopped hiccuping. This patient was my second one in Wigratzbad where I had only chronic patients for 11 years.

My first patient had been Mr. Joseph Rädler, who suffered from cancer of the large and small intestines. As you can see from the testimonial, he is the brother of Miss Antonie Rädler who owns the sanitarium. This man was seriously ill and unable to sit. After examining him, I assured him that after eight days he would be able to do some light work again because his heart and lungs were in extremely good condition. In fact, it took only five days until he could work again.

When the clergyman got well within five minutes, everyone trusted me completely and within three days I had advised more than 60 patients with great success. I believe that all the patients who suffer with hiccups will be very thankful to me. I would be very much obliged if they would inform me of their success in this respect.

Hypertension
see *Blood Pressure, Too High.*

Infertility
See *Childlessness*

Inflammations of Any Kind
If inflammation occurs, the kidneys are not functioning properly and therefore you should take *kidney tea for three weeks.* In addition, you should make up packs with diluted vinegar and place them on the affected parts. Foot packs (see *Circulation)* are also very effective, particularly in the case of *meningitis* and *inflammation of the eye.* Foot packs, like water-treading should only be done under the waning moon. This means you should start when the visible moon is on the decrease. It can be continued during the waxing moon (visible increase of the moon). (See also *Water Treatments.)*

In addition, you should drink a sip of pure water or sage tea every ten minutes. In all cases of inflammation you have to extinguish the "fire". Eating meat (especially pork or beef) and meat broth, or drinking alcohol (particularly white wine) is like trying to extinguish a fire by dousing it with gasoline.

Instead of making packs with diluted vinegar, you could make them with savoy cabbage leaves. They must be wrapped tightly to the affected area, securely attached and kept especially warm! You can leave such packs on for up to twelve hours, but never longer!

Inflammation of the Stomach

See *Stomach Disorders - (Gastritis).*

Influenza *(Grippe)*

In case of influenza, sponge the entire body every half hour with cold water using a moist towel. Half an hour after sponging for the sixth time, the patient should use Father Kneipp's short pack, leave it on for half an hour and remain in bed for another half hour without the pack. Then the patient should sponge all over with diluted vinegar, go to bed again, and remain there for four to six hours, covered lightly so as not to sweat again. After this time the patient should be well again, provided that he has followed my instructions properly.

Sponging the patient all over with a moist towel should only take two or three minutes. After every towel bath the patient should be wrapped up warmly, like a mummy. You should only be able to see the face. After the second, third or fourth sponge bath, the patient will sweat as if in a sauna.

If everyone followed this method when suffering from influenza, they would cut their health bills tremendously.

Take linden blossom (*Tilia europaea* or *Tilia cordata*), also called lime blossom, and elder blossom (or flower) tea (*Sambucus nigra*). Drink warm until you start to sweat, thereafter lukewarm. After that, drink Sage tea, orange juice and warm lemon juice.

People who eat a lot of beet root salad rarely get influenza. In February or March you should take one spoonful of buckthorn (*Rhamnus catharticus*) syrup or juice, for approximately three weeks, three times per day after each meal. This is one of the best ways of preventing influenza. If buckthorn juice is unavailable, take black currant juice or Schoenenberger Acerola Juice.

Insomnia

When suffering from insomnia, drink one or more cups of apple peel tea at night. This can be drunk warm or cold. The tea is a great tonic for the nerves and strengthens them considerably.

Because of the calming effect, I believe that there would never be any arguments within the family or with neighbors if everyone drank the tea at night. Apple peelings should be boiled for three to six minutes. If you prefer a sweeter taste then dried sugar cane juice or other unrefined sugar can be added.

If dried apple peelings are kept for 10 years, they will still have the same value as fresh ones. Apple peelings are never completely dry. They are always moist to the touch and never go grey.

Insufficient Bile
See *Bile.*

Jaundice
To treat jaundice, for four days eat nothing but black radish with the skins on and mashed potatoes without fat or salt but plenty of mixed-in black radish. The skin of the black radish is the most important part, therefore never peel this vegetable! In summer you will probably have to use other kinds of radish.

I once treated a case in which a woman had already had jaundice for three days and had not been to see a physician. I told her husband about my black radish treatment. However, she was unable to eat the black radish, so for four days she was given grated black radish peel with a little raw sugar added, and potato puree with black radish. After four days she did not look yellow any more and had no more discomfort.

Another case: Many years ago a man came to see me, bringing his father who had jaundice. It was late evening. At 10:00 p.m., I went into the garden with my flashlight and found two small black radishes, grated them right then and there and gave them to him to eat, together with a little raw sugar. As he wasn't very keen on black radish, it took him a while to get it down. As he was eating the second black radish and was just about to take another forkful, his cheeks suddenly turned red and, after a few days, the jaundice disappeared completely.

Kidney and Gall Bladder Attacks

For kidney and gall bladder colic I recommend a very hot horse-tail (*Equisetum arvense*) pack, which is left on for approximately half an hour. If the patient feels well with the pack on, it may be left on longer. After about twenty minutes, the pain will have decreased significantly.

Put a handful or more of horsetail inside a little sack and boil it for about 10 to 15 minutes.

Mental Disorder

See *Neurosis – Mental Disorder – Depression.*

Moth Spray

If you have naphthalene, man-made camphor from waste coal, DDT or similar poisons for moths, cockroaches or flies, or air fresheners in the toilet, etc., you ought to remove these poisons completely and afterwards burn incense of fragrant resin in your home once a day for two weeks. The incense is made from a resin which is collected by ants and which is stored in ant hills (*can be purchased in pharmacies*). Frankincense (church incense) is a good substitute.

Anyone who has the above poisons in the house will not be successful in healing any illnesses.

Instead of using naphthalene, man-made camphor, DDT etc. against insects, use natural materials, such a lavender, walnut leaves, hops, woodruff, wormwood, curd soap, tobacco, perfume or champhora. Natural camphor, or champhora, comes from wood shavings of the camphor tree and is not harmful.

A Small Experience Involving Moth Poison

In 1945 I was on holidays with my mother and sister. As usual, I had a few books on healing treatments with me so I could learn from them. I was especially interested in the iris diagnosis of the eye by Dr. Wirz. As I had read a few pages, I glanced at my sister and said, "Come over here for a minute and read for yourself about what Dr. Wirz says regarding the various moth poisons. If you have such things in your home, they should be thrown away because no illness can be healed in their presence." My mother then said, "We have always had moth balls, and no one has been ill yet in our family!" In reality, hardly a month went by when there wasn't a medical doctor visiting our house. My mother had suffered from foot and leg trouble since my birth, and my father was an alcoholic. Crying bitter tears, he had promised my sisters and myself on numerous occasions that he would give up drinking. However, Dr. Wirz's book said: Alcoholism is also an illness. An alcoholic may promise himself a hundred times that he will stop, and the slightest excuse, such as happiness or sadness, can start him off again. This was exactly the case with my father to the day he died. He was a first class stone-mason but he never had any money because of his drinking problem. Therefore, my mother got hardly any money from him and had to work as a laundress to feed five children.

After this talk with my mother and my sister about the moth poison mentioned in Dr. Wirz's book, I knew that we would have had a good father if there had not been any moth balls in our home! Were we poor, then, because of this poison? Was that the reason why I could not go to high school, which had always been my greatest wish? I tried to make up for it by buying as many books as my meager pocket money allowed for. Happiness for me meant learning from these books and from lectures I attended. My principle was then, and still is now, to make the best of my time and not waste it even though I am eighty-nine years old (1988). I pray to God every day, thanking him that I can work, learn, teach, and thereby help my fellow man!

Myocardial (*Heart Muscle*) Damage

For myocardial damage, take an arm bath (heart bath) every day for eight days. Put both arms into cold water for twenty seconds and rotate them similar to the motion of a water wheel. Without drying your arms, swing them back and forth for ten minutes, both simultaneously in the same direction. Thereafter, sit down immediately and place both hands flat on the table.

By means of the arm bath, and swinging the arms lightly for ten minutes, the arms fill up with blood. This may cause considerable pain, particularly in the tenth minute. Keeping this blood from the heart for ten minutes is a relaxation for the heart, just as if you had spent one month resting in a sanitarium. If this is done for eight days, it corresponds to eight months spent in a health clinic.

Myocardial damage can be recognized by the lunula or half-moon on your finger nails (that is, if you can see the half-moon shape). The lunulas should be nicely curved and rounded. But if there is a gap in the curve or it juts upwards like a peak, it means that you suffer from myocardial damage. When the blood pressure is very low, no half-moon can be seen. (See also *Blood Pressure*.)

Neuralgia *(Trigeminal)*

See *Trigeminal Neuralgia*

Neurosis – Mental Disorder – Depression

Apple peel tea can help to heal these illnesses as with insomnia (See *Insomnia*). In addition, patients should drink a half cup of cranesbill tea (herb Robert, *Geranium robertianum*) every day. Place a pinch of herb Robert into one half cup of hot water and steep for ten minutes. This tea can be taken for a whole year. Balm (*Melissa officinalis*) and Primrose tea (*Primula officinalis*) will also help.

Besides these remedies, washing the whole body with diluted vinegar and water has a miraculous effect if done properly. There are obviously cases where even these specific applications cannot help any more. (For more on washing with vinegar-water solution see *Influenza*.)

Operation – How to Prepare for Surgery

If the operation is not scheduled immediately, then three weeks before the date drink kidney tea and sage tea. You should drink sage tea every day of your life, but definitely before an operation. Do not drink any alcohol! After the operation the patient is advised, "Now breathe deeply." This is very important indeed. But you should practice this breathing beforehand, so you can do it on your own as soon as you come out of the anesthesia. (For breathing exercises see *Breathing Exercises*.)

In 1947, I had a gall bladder operation and did not come out of the anesthesia until the fourth day after the operation. The head physician had already given up on me, as he later told me himself. If I had not known about breathing exercises, and had not done them, I would have certainly died. These breathing exercises were so painful that the doctor said to me, "A thousand doctors would not have done them, had they been in your place," and then he asked me whether I smoked. I replied that I did not. To which he said that a smoker would not have had the energy to do these exercises. I would like to add that a non-smoker has a much greater chance of coming out of an operation alive than a smoker. So please, at least stop smoking before an operation, because after the operation it will be forbidden anyway.

Before an operation it would be important for a patient to have a biorhythm check done. This method was invented by Dr. Fliess and the Engineer, Hans Früh. The latter unfortunately died in January, 1974. Biorhythm calculations are done by Firma Max Münger, Angewandte Biorhythmic und Periodizitätsforschung (The Max Münger Company of Applied Biorhythm and Periodicity Research), Hauptstrasse 225, CH 9104 Waldstatt, Switzerland. Tel.: 071 51 39 51. I have calculated – after the fact – as many as a thousand operations whose outcome, good or bad, I already knew. In each case I ascertained that my biorhythm calculations coincided exactly with the true outcome of each operation. How wonderful, if a biorhythm chart were taken into consideration for every operation performed on a non-emergency basis. It would be a blessing for the patients and an advantage to the good reputation of the surgeon, because complications would rarely occur. (Of course, in a thousand operations, there is bound to be an exception, even in the case of a favorable biorhythm test.) A doctor who had operated on a man with stomach cancer according to my calculations, remarked to me, "Well, where would we be if we always had to check the biorhythm first?" I replied, "A lot further than we would be otherwise." I then gave him proof, including several reports from well-known doctors and clinics, which convinced him of the value of these calculations. Unfortunately, this doctor died shortly thereafter. That was several years ago. It is a pity that there are still physicians who laugh at this science without ever taking the trouble to research it first. It goes without saying that a person should not pronounce judgment on something he knows nothing about. Every transition (in the biorhythm) whether for the male rhythm or for the female rhythm, or the intellectual rhythm, periodic or semi-periodic day, is a danger sign for undergoing an operation because of possible embolism, thrombosis, bleeding or even death.

Phlebitis

This is an inflammation of the inner membrane of a vein. To heal phlebitis, make a cold vinegar and water pack. Mud packs made with vinegar and water also work well and quickly. Curd (quark) packs can also be recommended. These packs are best applied one to three times daily. In this way the patient will be relieved of pain after three to four days. Kidney tea should be drunk too, as with all other illnesses. In all types of inflammation it is important to sip a little pure water frequently during the day. If the veins of the leg are affected, bandage the leg starting at the toe and do a lot of walking. Be careful, because phlebitis can lead to thrombosis.

Pregnancy

The very first thing is to realize that this is not a disease state but a state of inner joy! Pregnant women often make the mistake of eating too rich and too much, inspired by their desire to give birth to a strong baby. This is wrong, particularly in the last two months. Such a baby can often cause difficult labor. If a child is overfed while in the womb, it usually is a finicky eater afterwards. In order to avoid complications during birth, every mother-to-be should sip one half cup of cold silver lady's mantle (*Alchemilla alpina*) and lady's mantle (*Alchemilla vulgaris*) tea per day, but no more than half a cup per day, otherwise the opposite effect will be achieved! A pinch of mixed silver mantle and lady's mantle should be allowed to steep in half a cup of hot water for

10 minutes. It is better to drink a tea which is a mixture of these two herbs although they can also be drunk separately.

Prostate

To treat prostate problems (including cancer of the prostate), sip one cup of cold tea made from the small flowered willow herb (*Epilobium parviflorum*) per day. A pinch of this herb should be allowed to steep for ten minutes in one cup of hot water. In addition, drink kidney tea for three weeks, as recommended with all other illnesses. Because in many cases the problem turns out to be cancer of the prostate, it is best to immediately start my "Total Cancer Treatment."

If a man can only pass water in drops, he will usually find that after three days of starting the above treatment he will be able to pass water normally again.

You should drink sage tea all of your life, especially during the juice treatment. If you intend to start my "Total Cancer Treatment" you should read the Part II of this book.

Pulmonary Tuberculosis

See *Bronchitis and Pulmonary Tuberculosis*.

Renal Colic

See *Kidney and Gall Bladder Attacks*.

Rheumatism

To treat any kind of rheumatism, drink kidney tea for three weeks as with all other illnesses. In this case, however, it is recommended to stop drinking the tea after three weeks, and two weeks later start drinking it again for another three weeks. In the case of rheumatism, the body contains too much uric acid which crystallizes when the patient catches a cold, causing pain in the joints, muscles etc. The cold is usually on one side. By this I mean that a draft, will only be felt on a certain part of the body.

In 1943, I became convinced that with almost every illness the kidneys are not functioning properly. This is especially true in the case of rheumatism. For this reason you should avoid eating meat, meat broth, beef and pork, and most certainly smoked meat for a while. Do not drink any alcohol. Good health comes from good drinking and eating habits.

Drinking sage tea (*Salvia officinalis*) is also very important. He who always drinks sage tea will not fall ill easily. Sage tea contains every enzyme for every gland in the body. As mentioned before, a Roman scientist once wrote, "Why die when there is sage in the garden?" I think sage tea is the most important of all teas.

The most important points to follow in life are:
 1. Never eat reheated food.
 2. Always drink sage tea.
 3. Keep no poisons in the house (such as naphthalene, camphor, fly spray, etc.) Where there are such poisons, hardly any illness can be cured. This is particularly true in the case of rheumatic complaints. (See also *Moth Poison.*)

Patients are often told to take mud baths, thermal baths etc., but they usually do not achieve the desired success. The reason for this is that these baths can only have a positive effect if the patient is drinking kidney tea at the same time. Before taking a mud bath, the patient should always take herbal tinctures for the heart (20-30 drops of valerian or hawthorn tincture).

Slipped Discs
Some years ago I would send patients suffering from this condition to Dr. S. whom I thought to be the best chiropractor and who never let me down. Then this practitioner moved away and I was forced to send my patients to another chiropractor. Because I was convinced that this problem could be treated painlessly, I studied the spinal cord every day for 10 years. Then, with the help of numerous books, I found the answer to this riddle. I did not have the opportunity to test my findings until two patients I had sent to the chiropractor came crying back to me and told me their troubles. One of the women said to me, "I have been there three times but I would rather die than go again because the pain was so

bad." The other woman said, "I do not feel exactly like dying, but I have been there twelve times with no results." Well, I just did not know what to do with these patients, so I explained to them that I had been studying the spinal cord for 10 years and believed that I had found out how to treat it painlessly. I said to them, "If you will agree, I will try it out on you." Both of them were ready to try. They said that they had nothing to lose. I then informed them that they were going to be test cases and that I was having reservations about trying the treatment. Luckily, it turned out to be a complete success. Within a few minutes I had helped the two women without causing pain, and they went home healthy. Since that day I have treated more than seven thousand patients suffering from back problems which the chiropractor didn't help – and all without pain. Out of a hundred patients only a few had to come back a second or third time. While using this treatment, I had the privilege of attending to many well-placed ladies and gentlemen (among them were court officials, a public prosecutor and his mother, several professors, the wife of a notary public, engineers, many clergymen, more than 50 nuns). A short while ago, I treated the mother of a medical doctor to whom I had shown my method; both were very impressed by my method, as was the wife of a medical doctor who was a chiropractor herself.

I do not believe that there is such a thing as a worn disc. As a point in case, I was treating a nun (who was only thirty years old), whose X-rays showed no discs left whatsoever. She had been told that she would have to spend the rest of her life in a plaster cast. In her case only three treatments were required. The first treatment was on January 9, 1970, the second three days later, and the third eight days after that. As a result of the three treatments she is healthy, works in the kitchen, and has now been sent to Columbia for a few years. Another nun from Yugoslavia, who is in France now, also received three treatments from me. She previously had undergone surgery of the spine and had six to eight artificial vertebrae made of silver. For two and a half years she had been bed-ridden in a plaster cast and was told that she would spend the rest of her life in a wheel chair. After the first treatment she was playing tag with the children outside my house. She also carried a small child in her arms. Her sister, the wife of an engineer and mother of a medical doctor, who was with me in the room, saw this and tears of happiness came to her eyes. Her brother-in-law, Mr. W.W., was present and was very moved as well. That was years ago. This nun came to visit me with her sister and brother-in-law a year after the treatment. When she told me that she felt healthy and had experienced no recurrences, it was a great joy for me.

I would now like to explain from my experience, how I envision damaged discs. In my opinion, the discs do not wear out, but only get pressed together and dry out. For example: Imagine a sponge measuring 50 cm x 50 cm x 50 cm. Place a heavy weight on this sponge of approximately 50 kilograms. It will then be pressed into a thin plate. If you leave this weight for six weeks and then take it off, the sponge will stay pressed together like a thin plate. But, if you pour water on this sponge, it will become approximately 50 centimeters high again.

What I do, then, is analogous to the example of the sponge. First, using my sense of touch, I painlessly stretch the spine downwards at the sacrum (two to five times, depending on the strength of the person) until I feel the spine relaxing and stretching. Then I place St. John's wort oil (*Hypericum perforatum*) over it and this works exactly like water on a sponge. It is equivalent to taking the weight off the sponge. Because the spine is stretched, the oil can penetrate all the way to the discs which then open up, like the sponge rising again after water is poured on it. At this point the slipped disc can be put back into place without causing any pain.

I would like to give you one more example. If a chain is pulled tight, then none of the links can be moved. If the chain is loose, then they can all be moved. When the spinal cord regains its full mobility through the oil, then the nerves are not trapped any longer, and the patient is well again. Without previous stretching, the St. John's wort oil has no effect.

What will physicians and chiropractors say about my discovery and my explanations regarding this matter? Some will be pleased to have found a method which is painless and in which an X-ray is not required. Others will say that this method is too quick and too inexpensive. In my opinion, though, medical doctors should be there to serve their patients – and not the other way around.

Smoking is Harmful

People who realize just how harmful smoking is, do not smoke. Nowadays, smoking is even more destructive than before because we are breathing in more harmful air. I would say that smoking one cigarette today is the equivalent of smoking three in the past. If you smoke 10 or 20 cigarettes per day you are greatly damaging your health.

What is even worse, the lungs are affected. Notice how smokers cough in the morning and what they discharge. Now consider cancer of the lungs. Non-smokers rarely suffer from this disease. How many smokers have cancer of the larynx? Moreover, smoking harms the stomach, regardless of whether a smoker inhales or not. If a non-smoker has to undergo surgery, his chances of survival are much greater than those of a smoker. This is also true for accident victims. By the way, aside from accident victims, most leg amputations have to be performed on smokers.

In order to give up smoking, do the following: Smoke, and enjoy a cigarette, and say firmly to yourself: "I am not going to smoke anymore." Think of all the disadvantages of smoking and how much money you would spend in 10, 20 or 30 years. If everyone had to buy cigarettes for the whole year on January 1st, there would be a lot fewer people who smoke. It is much more dangerous for women to smoke and, if they are pregnant, smoking endangers both mother and child!

Smoking has many, many disadvantages and absolutely no advantages.

Many people will say that they know somebody who has smoked since he was young and who has lived for a long time. Well, that may be so, but if two people do the same thing, it is not necessarily the same for both. Besides, people may be able to reach an age of more than a hundred! Each animal lives seven times as long as its development requires, unless it is killed, and human beings are not fully developed before the age of 20 or 21.

Sores (open)

See *Ulcers (Exterior)*.

Sore Throat

To treat the pain, gargle with sage tea, alternating with pimpernel (*Pimpinella magna*) tea. The first tablespoonful is gargled and spat out, the same happens with the second spoonful; with the third you still gargle but this time you swallow the tea (as with diptheria). Sage tea is left to steep for 10 minutes in hot water. To prepare pimpernel tea, put one teaspoonful in one quarter liter (1 cup/250 ml) of water and boil for three minutes.

If suffering from strep throat combined with a high fever (*streptococcus*), you should seek the advice of your physician to prevent possible permanent health damage.

The most effective method of treating a sore throat is a potato pack placed around the neck. Boil three egg-sized potatoes until they are soft. Place the boiled potatoes on a clean linen cloth, cover them and mash them with your hands or a roller. Then apply the poultice to your neck as hot as you can stand it. Tie a warm scarf over it, put on a woolen hat and rest in bed **on your back**, making sure that you are well covered, especially that your arms and shoulders are under the blankets. Leave the potato pack in place for two hours. Do not worry if you fall asleep during this time; you can simply leave it on until you wake up.

Stomach Disorders
Gastritis

In case of gastritis, when the pain is at its worst (which is usually before meals) take a cup of warm water which has been boiled six times. (This means boil, cool, boil again, cool again and so on, six times.) After drinking this water, the patient will burp continuously for some time. After each burp, there is a feeling of relief. About five minutes later, the patient feels fine and will hardly ever have trouble again. In the days when people did not cook with electric heat, the warm water was taken from a water basin which was installed in every wood-burning stove. I suffered from this illness myself for three years before I knew much about natural healing. A good lady, which I met on my way when the pain was at its worst, told me what to do. I followed her instructions and, after five minutes, I was cured of this terrible illness. Even today I am very much obliged to this woman, Mrs. Angelina Nikolussi.

Heartburn

People who suffer from heartburn have too much gastric acid. A remedy for this condition is wormwood tea (*Artemisia absinthium*) (See *Other Stomach Disorders*). For immediate relief, eat a piece of fatty cheese (as long as the liver and gall bladder are functioning normally) **without** bread.

Cheese with a high fat content absorbs the excess gastric acid. Eaten with bread, however, it produces even more gastric acid and the heartburn gets worse.

Ulcers (Gastric and Duodenal)

If the liver and gall bladder are in order then, for two days eat only whipped cream with plenty of honey, dried sugar cane juice or other unrefined sugar and nothing else. Do not drink anything during these two days, not even tea or milk. On the third day, drink camomile tea, sage tea or mallow leaf tea (*Malva silvestris*) taken from a spoon. You can then begin to eat normally as the ulcers should be gone.

If, however, the liver and gall bladder are not in good order, never try the fresh whipped cream diet. In such cases, daily sip one half to two cups of cold mallow leaf tea (*Malva silvestris*). The mallow should be left to steep in hot water for 10 minutes. The patients in question will probably have to drink this tea for a whole year. (Note: If you want to avoid dairy you can use flax seeds; two tablespoons soaked overnight in 1/4 liter of water (250 ml) sweetened as above are extremely beneficial for stomach ulcers.) Remember stomach ulcers can lead to cancer.

Other Stomach Disorders

There are, of course, many different stomach complaints, and not all of them can be treated in the same way. But very often it helps to take one half cup of cold wormwood tea (*Artemisia absinthium*) daily, sipping it by the spoonful.

Wormwood tea is usually made too strong. To prepare it correctly, take a small pinch of wormwood and let it steep in one half cup of hot water – but for only three seconds. In other words, put a small pinch of wormwood into a tea strainer and submerge into the hot water pressing down with a teaspoon for just three seconds (say "a hundred and one three times). Thereafter the tea should be ready. Finished wormwood tea should not look any different than pure water.

In case of *stomach poisoning* the wormwood should be boiled for two to three minutes (or allowed to steep for 10 minutes in hot water). However, after two to three days of drinking it this way, it should again be steeped for only **three seconds**, as previously described. The patient should continue to drink the tea for about 10 to 14 days.

Surprisingly, cold point-packs can often be remedial for many stomach illnesses. Packs are at first made with a solution of water and vinegar and after two to three days with normal cold water. To prepare a point-pack, take a large folded handkerchief (or linen cloth). Make it damp (not wet). Then apply the damp handkerchief to the stomach region and wrap up completely in warm towels or blankets.

Stuttering

This speech impediment is a nervous disorder. The patient should drink one half to one and a half cups of warm or cold apple peel tea at night, as well as one half cup of balm mint (*Melissa officinalis*) tea. Apple peels must be boiled for three to six minutes. Those who prefer the tea sweet can sweeten it with some dried sugar cane juice or other unrefined sugar.

However, stuttering can also be caused by cramping in the brain. If a person who stammers wants to talk, his nerves become cramped so that he is hardly able to utter a word. To treat this, he should drink a quarter liter (1 cup/250 ml) of milk with cinquefoil (*Potentilla anserina*) in the morning. Those who cannot tolerate milk, can boil a pinch of cinquefoil in wine or cider. (See also *Cramps*).

Surgery

See *Operation, How to Prepare For.*

Teething Pains

Sometimes babies experience great pain when their teeth emerge and they cry for days. This can be easily remedied by giving them a teaspoonful of pure water every ten minutes. As soon as a crying baby gets a teaspoonful of water in his mouth, he will stop crying immediately. Ten minutes later he will usually become restless again, so give him another spoonful of water.

If you do this, your child will never have trouble teething and the teeth he gets will be better and stronger than they would have been otherwise.

Throat

See *Sore Throat*

Tinnitus

See *Buzzing of the Ears*

Trigeminal Neuralgia

With this extremely painful illness, relief can be obtained by a light pounding massage which is done with a new collapsible ten-piece wooden carpenter's rule, 200 cm in length (diagram 1). Unfold the rule to its full length, then fold into a V-shape at the center (diagram 2). Now fold the upper sections of the V down, so that it looks like a big M (diagram 3). Push the M together (diagram 4) then fold the upper four sections again at the 20 cm mark (diagram 5). Now you can begin the massage. Hold the meter-rule with one hand approximately at the 93 centimeter mark (see diagram 6). The piece that should lightly pound the upper forehead should be approximately at the eight centimeter mark (see diagram 7). If the rule is properly folded, the pounding results in a light double hit which does not hurt at all. Do not use the upper end, though, (at the 12 to 18 centimeter mark) because that could hurt. After each 'hit' the neuralgic pain lessens, and after five to 10 minutes there is no more pain at all. After 12 to 24 hours the pain could return but not as strongly. In this case, repeat the massage for ten days, again for five to 10 minutes daily. There will soon be a marked improvement.

There are people suffering from trigeminal neuralgia who do not wash their faces for days on end because they can already feel the pain when their hands are only near their faces. I can console those people and reassure them that this massage, properly applied, does not hurt.

Through the pounding movement, the electromagnetic iron particles located around the trigeminus are separated demagnetized, and easily transferred into the blood stream.

In addition, breathing exercises will be highly beneficial, as in the case of very high blood pressure. (see *Breathing Exercises.*)

[*Editorial*: Instead of a 200 centimeter long meter-rule, logically you can also use a 100 centimeter, six part folding meter-rule. The effect will be the same.]

Tuberculosis *(Lung)*
See *Bronchitis and Pulmonary Tuberculosis.*

Ulcers, (Gastric and Duodenal)
See *Stomach Disorders*

Ulcers (Exterior)

To treat exterior ulcers, prepare a fresh whipping cream pack with a lot of sugar added. The cream cools and softens, the sugar heals the ulcer. Instead of whipping cream, bee honey can be put on an ulcer.

Vaginal Discharge (White, Yellow and Brown)

To treat white discharge, every hour take a small sip of tea made from the white dead nettle blossoms (*Lamium album*) until everything has cleared up. To prepare, take a **small** pinch of dead nettle and steep in a half cup of hot water for 10 minutes.

To treat yellow and brown discharge, every hour take a small sip of tea made from silver lady's mantle (*Alchemilla alpina*) and lady's mantle (*Alchemilla vulgaris*) together with a pinch of yellow or white dead nettle blossoms. Put a pinch of mixed herbs into half a cup of hot water and steep for 10 minutes. The tea is to be taken cold.

Make sure to add dead nettle blossoms equal to the amount of the other two herbs combined, about 20 to 30 nettle blossoms.

Drinking more than half a cup of this tea per day would do more harm than good.

Varicose Ulcers

To treat varicose ulcers, take a full bath with horsetail (*Equisetum arvense*) extract daily for two weeks. Stay in the bath for half an hour. To prepare the bath, put the horsetail into a linen cloth and boil for 10 to 15 minutes. Also drink kidney tea for three weeks and drink sage tea as suggested with all ailments. Varicose ulcers should be treated with horsetail baths only. Any other baths would not be advised in this case. Before starting the bath, take heart drops (see *Rheumatism*). After the bath, bandage your legs and walk a lot!

Alpine horsetail contains 96 per cent silicic acid, the tall and coarse kind approximately 40 per cent and the small and coarse type which often grows in potato fields, only 16 per cent. If only 16 per cent horsetail is available, then more has to be added to the bath.

Varicose Veins of the Legs

If you suffer from this complaint, you should lie on your back several times a day. Raise your right leg, wait five to eight seconds, shake your leg, wait another five to eight seconds and then lower your leg again. After resting for five to eight seconds, repeat the exercise with the left leg. Thereafter do the exercise with both legs at the same time. After lowering both legs, do not get up until all the blood has flowed back into the legs, that is, after about 40 to 60 seconds. The more often you do this during the day, the sooner the varicose veins will disappear.

The process can be explained as follows: When the legs are raised and left in the air for 10 to 16 seconds, all the blood flows downward, and the veins are left with little blood. If the legs are then lowered, fresh blood flows into the blood vessels, nourishing, reviving, and contracting them.

Varicose veins are caused by the muscles of the veins becoming slack (as if paralyzed) and thus becoming enlarged. To make a comparison: If an inner bicycle tube has a weak spot and is pumped up, the tube will balloon out at that point just as varicose veins do.

Warts and Birthmarks

These growths can sometimes be non-malignant forms of cancer. They are easily treated. Simply cover the affected area with marigold leaves or blossoms (*Calendula officinalis*), or both. Bind a tight-fitting cloth around it, and leave on overnight. If marigolds are not available, you can also use marigold ointment (calendula cream).

Avoid operations on birthmarks. Any surgery on birthmarks can be very dangerous!

Water Treatments

Water-treading

Water-treading as well as *alternating foot baths* (see below) should always be started in the phase of the waning (decreasing) moon (that is, when the moon is in the signs of Cancer, Leo, Virgo, Libra or Scorpio). If, for example, a woman starts the water-treading during the waxing (growing) moon (that is, when the moon is in Capricorn, Aquarius, Pisces, Aries or Taurus), then the blood will rush to her head instead of her feet. I read this in an old book and have experienced the truth of it over and over again. You can look up the moon's phases in a farmer's almanac and in some calendars.

Water-treading is done the following way: At the start, the feet should be warm, the stomach never full. Walk for 20 minutes before and after water-treading; before, to get the feet warm; after, to get the feet warm again. Water-treading is done in cold water, so if you stand around or, worse yet, sit down afterwards instead of walking, your feet will get even colder than before. You would have to do at least ten proper sessions of water-treading before the damage done could be repaired. Water-treading means walking in cold water while the feet are alternately lifted as high as possible, going air-water, air-water, etc. A bathtub is a good place for this therapy. In each session, first tread water that reaches just above the ankle, for five to six minutes; then tread water that reaches below the knee, for only three to four minutes. Water-treading is really helpful when there is not enough circulation to the feet.

Alternating Baths (feet and arms)

An *alternating foot bath* should be started only in the moon's waning phase (see *Water-treading*). Here are the instructions: At the start, the feet should always be warm and the stomach never full. Whether you do a foot or an arm bath, you should always put the right foot (or the right arm) into the warm or cold water first. That is why three different buckets are required for an alternating foot bath: one basin containing warm water in the middle and one on each side containing cold water. Sit on a chair and put your feet in the warm water, which should be at a temperature of 28 to 30 Celsius (82.5 to 86 F). For the next ten minutes, keep pouring in more hot water until the temperature reaches 40 to 45 Celsius (104 to 113 F). In the end, the warm water should reach up to the middle of your calves (as should the cold water). Now put your right foot into the cold water on the right, and then put your left foot into the cold water on the left. Put the right foot back in the warm water, then put the left foot back, and so on, repeating the cycle over and over. Each time, the feet should stay in the cold water for three to four seconds and in the warm water for five to six seconds. Because of this alternating action, the warm water gets gradually cooler and the cold water gets warmer. If the feet are numb, it is advisable to keep alternating until warm and cold water are the same temperature. After such a bath, lie down for half an hour covered with a blanket. *Alternating foot baths* alleviate problems of circulation, such as cold or numb feet. They also help if there are problems with menstruation.

An *alternating arm bath* can be taken at any phase of the moon. It is done exactly the same way as a foot bath, except that only two basins are needed here. The water should be deep enough to reach the middle of the upper arms. A story told by Mr. Karl Zerlauth will illustrate the amazing effects of alternating baths.

He knew a man whose fingers on the left hand became numb, then the whole hand, and eventually his forearm up to the elbow. He went to his medical doctor who advised him to have the arm amputated immediately. The doctor believed that if this condition was allowed to continue, it would lead to the man's death. This man then went to the hospital and the doctors wanted to keep him there to perform the amputation the very next day. As this man was a farmer and was suffering no pain, he said, "Why keep me here? I'll go home and be back here at 6:00 a.m. with an empty stomach." So they let him go. The next morning, on his way to the hospital, he met Mr. Karl Zerlauth, the Director of the Kneipp-Spa Center in Austria, who was on his early morning walk.

Mr. Zerlauth greeted this man in a friendly manner because he knew him quite well. But the man returned the greeting in a subdued and depressed way. So Mr. Zerlauth asked him why he was so sad. The farmer told him the whole story. Mr. Zerlauth replied, "Chin up, because you won't need to have an operation. Turn around, go home and try alternating baths." The farmer replied, "But I have promised the hospital that I would arrive punctually, and I can't keep the doctors waiting." Now Mr. Zerlauth (from whom I have learned so much!) in his great wisdom said, "If there were a hundred doctors waiting, there would be nothing as important as saving your arm." The farmer then followed his advice, went home and tried the arm bath until both basins of water had reached the same temperature. It was a full success. He regained normal feeling in his fingers. He took another two arm baths and, that evening, a

99

third – whereupon the feeling in his whole arm returned. He was healed. You can well imagine how happy this man was, and I am also very happy and thankful to Mr. Karl Zerlauth, for telling me this story, from which I have learned a lot.

Water Veins – Also Called Earth Rays *(Ground Radiation)*

It has been my experience that most cancer patients and others suffering from seemingly incurable diseases, are sleeping on top of so-called damaging earth rays which are even more dangerous where they cross.

If this is suspected, get in touch with a water diviner who works with a divining rod or a pendulum to look for these veins in your house, and then move your bed if necessary to sleep where the ground is clear of radiation. There are people who do not believe this, but if you ask six water diviners to visit you and each finds the water veins in the same spot, then it must be true. In my house, for example, a divining rod does not move, but this does not mean that ground radiation does not exist. There are people who are healthy and who move to a different house, and from that day onwards are always ill. This is only because now they are sleeping on a water vein. There are several books which are rich in evidence about this fact and which would convince you that this is the truth.

[Editorial: A good book available on this subject is entitled: "Earth Currents, a Causative Factor of Cancer and Other Diseases," by Gustav Freiherr von Pohl, Frech Verlag. This books is most difficult to obtain in health food stores and book stores. You may be able to obtain it by writing directly to *alive* **Books**, Vancouver, BC Canada.]

Why Reheated Food May Be Worthless

When a person becomes hungry, it is a sign that cells have died which have to be replaced by eating fresh food. In reheated food, not too many vitamins are left, so these cells cannot be replaced properly.

Reheated food is, therefore, worthless and in certain circumstances even dangerous.

Reheated food is nothing but useless ballast, not capable of nourishing the body. Such food fills up holes and quells hunger, but man cannot exist on it. Convenience food such as TV dinners and other precooked meals should also be viewed as reheated food.

Some people may say that they eat fresh food besides reheated food. I can only say to them that in this way not all cells which are dying every day can be replaced. This can be compared to a tiled roof. If a storm rips 10 tiles from a roof and these are replaced with only eight tiles, and if after the next storm another 10 tiles are replaced with only eight, one will soon find oneself without a roof over one's head.

I could quote many more examples regarding people who have eaten a lot of reheated food. Therefore, remember: never again eat reheated food!

RESOURCES

SOURCES FOR INGREDIENTS

Many health foods stores supply herbs and juices. If you are having difficulty finding supplies, the following companies may supply ingredients by mail order or will direct you to your local supplier. Before starting the fast, make sure you have enough supplies on hand to last for 42 days. You do not want to go through 21 days of fasting only to find out that you cannot continue because your store ran out of the juices or teas you need.

IN CANADA:

Supplier of the Biotta Organic Juices and Breuss Vegetable Juice:
Bioforce Canada Inc.
1111 Gorham, unit 9
Newmarket, ON
L3Y 7V1 Canada
Toll-free: 1-800-264-5588
Fax: 905-853-1527 or
66 Brunswick
Dollard-des-Ormeaux,
Quebec
H9B 2L3 Canada
Tel: 514-421-3441
Toll-free: 1-800-361-6320
Fax: 514-421-6446
www.bioforce.com
info@Bioforce.ca

Supplier of Cranesbill (Herb Robert) Tea, organic cellular plant juices (including black radish juice):
Flora Manufacturing & Distributing Ltd.
7400 Fraser Park Drive
Burnaby, BC V5J 5B9
Canada
Tel: 604-436-6000
www.florahealth.com
Toll-free: 888-436-6697

Supplier of herbs and teas:
Puresource Inc.
7018 Wellington Rd
124 South
Guelph, Ontario
N1H 6J4 Canada
Tel: 519-837-2140
Toll-free: 1-800-265-7245
Fax: 1-519-837-1584

Supplier of the therapeutical Greenstar juicer:
Alpha Health Products Ltd.
7434 Fraser Park Dr.
Burnaby, BC
V5J 5B9 Canada
800-663-2212 or
604-436-0545
www.alphahealth.ca

IN USA:

Flora Inc.
PO Box 73,
805 East Badger
Lynden, WA 98264 USA
Tel: 360-354-2110
www.florahealth.com

Supplier of Biotta lacto-fermented vegetable juices and the Breuss Vegetable Juice:
Rapunzel Pure Organics Inc.
2424 State Route 203
Valatie, NY 12184 USA
800-207-2814
518-392-8620
info@rapunzel.com
www.rapunzel.com

Supplier of herb tinctures:
Herb Pharm
PO Box 116
Williams, OR 97544 USA
Tel: 514-846-6262
Toll-free: 800-348-4372
info@herb-pharm.com
www.herb-pharm.com

Supplier of herbs:
Blessed Herbs
109 Barre Plains Road
Oakham, MA 01068
USA
Tel: 508-882-3839
Toll-free: 1-800-489-4372
blessed-herbs@blessedherbs.com
www.blessedherbs.com

GERMANY

Manufacturer of Eden juices:
Eden Waren GMBH Export
Lüner Rennbahn 18
21339 Lüneburg,
Germany
Tel: -49-4131-98506
Fax: -49-4131-985300
E-Mail: info@eden.de
www.eden.de

SWITZERLAND

Supplier of the Breuss Vegetable Juice, and lacto-fermented juices:
Biotta AG
Planzbergstrasse 8
Postfach
CH-8274 Tägerwilen,
Switzerland
Tel: 41 (0) 71 666 80 80
Fax: +41 (0) 71 666 80 81
e-mail: info@biotta.ch
www.biotta.ch

HELPFUL HINTS FOR JUICES AND TEAS

About juice: If you make your own juice, find a supplier of organic fruits and vegetables that can supply what you need for the coming six weeks. If you use bottled juices and mix them yourself, buy 12 half-litre bottles each of beet, carrot and celeriac juice and six small bottles of black radish juice. If you use the Breuss juice from Biotta, order three cases or 36 half-litre bottles from a retailer or distributor. At the rate of one tablespoon of juice every fifteen minutes to half an hour, you will not finish a whole bottle each day. Remember the juice is not only for the fast but also it makes a nice addition to your diet after the fast is over. When you drink the juice, it is difficult to fill a tablespoon without spilling and sip the juice gradually and slowly. For this reason, it helps to use a small glass, such as a shot or liqueur glass. Now you can sit down with your juice and sip it at your leisure.

About teas: For the kidney tea, the quantities given in Breuss' recipe are sufficient for the time the tea must be taken. For the cranesbill tea (herb Robert, *Geranium robertianum),* get one 85g package. For the sage tea with its additions of St. John's wort, peppermint and balm mint, buy two 85g packages of each. You need to prepare and drink about three litres of sage tea every day to replace lost body fluids. It is advisable to get a thermos bottle so you can carry your tea with you. If you do not finish your packages of sage tea and additional teas, remember Breuss recommends drinking sage tea "for the rest of your life".

About onion broth: It is vital to have a ready supply of organic onions for the duration of the fast. The safest way to ensure this supply is to buy approximately 84 lemon-sized onions and store them in a cool dark place. For the broth, try to find vegetable cubes that do not have added peanut fats or extra protein. Read the labels! A good broth to use is BMB, Dr. Bronner's Balanced Mineral Broth, a concentrated vegetable broth available in many health food stores. You will need approximately three 474 ml (1 pint) bottles for the fast.

BREUSS FASTING CLINIC

The authentic Breuss Cancer Treatment is offered with medical care and supervision in a clinic in Germany.

Breuss Fasting Clinic
Kurhotel Chattenbühl
An der Rehbocksweide 29 a
34346 Hannoversch Münden
Germany
Tel: -49-554133461
Fax: -49-554131086

Breuss Cancer Care Program
Designed for those who wish to have personal and educational assistance to lead them through the Breuss fast.
Fresh made juices and herbal tea preparations are provided.
Includes nutritional counseling, as well as resource materials.
Comfortable accommodations for three to five weeks in private home with serene surroundings.
7528 Lambeth Drive
Burnaby, BC, Canada   V5E 1Z4
Tel: 604-521-0659

For this book in other languages contact:
Walter Margreiter
Im Hag 23
A-6714 Nüziders, Austria
Tel: -43-55-526-4290

NOTES

RECOMMENDED READING

BOOKS:

How I Cured Myself of Cancer by Howard Wagar, Self-Publisher, out of print
This easy to read booklet tells the story of the author's fight against the effects
of cobalt treatment and surgery for cancer of the lymph glands.

Cancer Therapy by Max Gerson, The Gerson Institute, San Diego CA, USA
www.gerson.org. A review of fifty cancer cases and their cure by diet therapy.

Cancer Therapy by Ralph Moss, Equinox, Brooklyn NY, USA
One hundred non-toxic or less-toxic treatments for cancer.

The Essiac Report by Richard Thomas, Alternative Treatment Info. Network,
Los Angeles CA, USA . The complete facts about Essiac, an incredibly effective herbal cancer remedy.

How to Get Well by Paavo Airola, Health Plus, Phoenix AZ, USA
The most practical and authoritative manual on proven and effective
drugless treatments.

What Your Doctor Won't Tell You by Jane Heimlich, Harper Collins Canada
A survey of the latest nonconventional medical treatments for
today's most prevalent diseases.

Prescription for Nutritional Healing by Phyllis and James Balch, Avery,
Garden City Park NY, USA. A complete and authoritative guide to dealing
with health disorders through nutritional, herbal and supplemental therapies.

The Oil-Protein Diet Cookbook by Johanna Budwig, Apple, Vancouver BC
Canada. Good fats in balance with protein, prepared in many variations.

Healing with Herbal Juices by Siegfried Gursche, Alive, Vancouver BC
Canada, out of print. A practical guide to herbal juice therapy: nature's preventative medicine.

Juicing — for the health of it! by Siegfried Gursche, Alive Publishing Group,
Vancouver, BC Canada

All of these books are available at your local bookstore or health
food store.

MAGAZINES AND PERIODICALS:

alive
Canada's #1-Read Magazine of
Natural Health
7432 Fraser Park drive
Burnaby BC   V5J 5B9 Canada
Tel: 604-435-1919
Toll Free: 800-663-6580
Fax: 604-435-4888
Toll Free Fax: 800-663-6597
www.alive.com
Canada's leading consumer publication designed for people interested in natural health. Features short, educational and up-to-date articles on current and relevant issues written by health professionals and personalities.

Townsend Letter for Doctors
and Patients
911 Tyler Street
Port Townsend WA   98368-6541
360-385-6021
Fax 360-385-0699
www.tldp.com

An Examiner of Medical
Alternatives
Herbalgram
PO Box 144345
Austin TX   78714-4345
512-926-4900
Fax 512-926-2345
www.herbalgram.com
Published by the American Botanical Council and the Herb Research Foundation, this magazine is an educational tool for anyone interested in the healing potential of plants and herbs.

The Cancer Chronicles
Toll Free: 800-980-1234
www.ralphmoss.com
An electronic publication that gives serious consideration to alternative treatments for cancer. Has reports on over 200 different types of cancer.

Felix Letter
PO Box 7094
Berkeley CA   94707
An educational publication discussing nutrition and healthy eating habits.

List of Herbs
(English/Latin/German)

Angelica	*Angelica archangelica*	Engelwurz
Balm Mint	*Melissa officinalis*	Melisse/Zitronenkraut
Bloodroot - see Tormentil		
Buckthorn	*Rhamnus catharticus*	Kreuzdorn
Calendula - see Marigold		
Camomile	*Anthemis nobilis*	Kamille
Camphor (Natural)	*Cinnamomum camphora*	Kampferbaum
Celandine	*Chelidonium majus*	Schöllkraut
Centaury	*Centaurium minus*	Tausendguldenkraut
Chickweed	*Stellaria media*	Hühnerdarm
Cinquefoil/Silverweed	*Potentilla anserina*	Fingerkraut
Cinquefoil	*Potentilla recta*	Hohes Fingerkraut
Cranesbill/Red Cranesbill (herb Robert)	*Geranium robertianum*	Storchenschnabelkraut
Dandelion	*Taraxacum officinale*	Löwenzahn
Dead/Blind Nettle (white)	*Lamium album*	Weisse Taubnessel
Elder	*Sambucus nigra*	Holunder/Schwarzer
Eyebright	*Euphrasia rostkoviana*	Augentrost
Ground Ivy	*Glechoma hederaceum*	Gundelrebe
Hawthorn	*Crataegus oxyacantha*	Weissdorn
Herb Bennet/Wood Avens	*Geum urbanum*	Echte Nelkenwurz
Herb Robert – See Cranesbill/Red Cranesbill		
Hop	*Humulus lupulus*	Hopfen
Horsetail	*Equisetum arvense*	Katzenschwanz
Houseleek	*Sempervivum tectorum*	Hauswurz
Iceland Moss	*Cetraria islandica*	Isländisches Moos
Kidney Vetch	*Anthyllis vulneraria*	Wundklee
Knot Grass	*Polygonum aviculare*	Vogelknöterich
Lady's Mantle	*Alchemilla vulgaris*	Frauenmantel
Linden	*Tilia europaea*	Linde
Lungwort	*Pulmonaria officinalis*	Lungenkraut
Mallow	*Malva sylvestris*	Wilde Malve
Marigold	*Calendula officinalis*	Ringelblume

List of Herbs

Masterwort	*Peucedanum*	Meisterwurz
Meum mutellina	*Meum mutellina*	Muttern/Mataun
Milfoil/Yarrow	*Achillea millefolium*	Schafgarbe
Mistletoe	*Viscum album*	Mistel
Mullein	*Verbascum thapsiforme*	Grosse Königskerze
Nettle, Stinging	*Urtica dioica*	Brennessel
Pimpernel (great)	*Pimpinella magna*	Bibernelle
Pimpernel (small)	*Pimpinella saxifraga*	Kleine Bibernelle
Plantain (ribwort or pointed)	*Plantago lanceolata*	Spitzwegerich
Plantain (great or broad-leaved)	*Plantago major*	Breitblätterriger Wegerich
Primrose	*Primula veris*	Schlüsselblume
Ribwort – see Plantain		
Sage	*Salvia officinalis*	Salbei
St. John's wort	*Hypericum perforatum*	Johanniskraut
Silvery Lady's Mantle	*Alchemilla alpina*	Silbermantele
Tormentil	*Potentilla tormentilla*	Blutwurz
Valerian	*Valeriana officinalis*	Baldrian
Willow herb	*Epilobium angustifolium*	Weidenröschen
Woodruff	*Asperula odorata*	Wald Meister
Wormwood	*Artemisia absinthium*	Wermut

Index

A

Abdominal dropsy, 57, 72
Adrenal gland, 57
Agoraphobia, 57, 68
Alcohol, 55, 71, 73, 78, 83, 87
Alcoholism, 57, 82
Anemia, 58, 73-74
Appetite, 3, 59
Arteriosclerosis, 59-60
Arthritis, 7, 33-34, 60
Arthrosis, 34, 60
Asthma, 60

B

Bad breath, 61
Basedow's disease, 61, 75
Bed-wetting, 61
Bile, 62, 75, 80
Bilious colic, 62
Birthmarks, 62, 97
Bleeding of any kind, 59, 62
Breathing exercises, 57-58, 61,
    63-65, 84, 95
Bronchitis, 65, 69, 86, 95
Buzzing of the ears, 65, 94

C

Cataracts, 66
Chilblains, 66
Circulatory disorders, 61, 67
Claustrophobia, 57, 68
Colic, 62, 68, 81, 86
Constipation, 38, 68
Convulsions, 68
Coughs, 19, 69

Cramps, 60, 69, 94
Cranesbill tea, 24, 31, 37-38,
    57, 67, 83, 103
Crooked fingers, 70

D

Depression, 45, 47, 71, 81, 83
Diabetes, 31, 35, 58, 71
Diphtheria, 39, 71
Discs, 18, 29, 76, 87-89
Dropsy of the heart, 72
Duodenal, 73, 92, 95
Dysentery, 62, 71, 73

F,G

Fainting, 73-75
Gastritis, 62, 75, 79, 91
Goiter, 61, 75
Ground radiation, 43, 100

H

Hay fever, 76
Headaches, 5, 17, 76
Heartburn, 92
Hemorrhoids, 77
Hiccups, 77-78
High blood pressure, 63, 95
Hypochondriacs, 54, 56

I,J

Infertility, 67, 78
Inflammations, 30, 78
Influenza, 75, 79, 83
Insomnia, 79, 83
Jaundice, 80

K,L

Kidney tea, 30, 33, 37-38, 42, 47, 52-53, 66, 72, 78, 83, 85-87, 96, 103-104
Leukemia, 7, 22, 27, 45-101
Low blood pressure, 63-64

M,N

Mental disorders, 71, 81, 83
Myocardial damage, 77, 82-83
Naphthalene, 48-52, 60, 81, 87
Neurosis, 71, 81, 83
Non-toxic insect repellents, 81

O,P

Onion broth, 23, 35-36, 103
Operations, 2-4, 6-9, 17, 24, 26, 42, 50, 54, 56, 83-85, 94, 99
Phlebitis, 85
Pregnancy, 85
Prostate, 41, 66, 86

R,S

Radiation, 2, 6, 8, 11, 31, 35, 37, 42-43, 100
Reheated food, 66, 87, 100-101
Renal colic, 86
Rheumatism, 60, 70, 86-87, 96

Sage tea, 16-17, 24, 29-31, 33, 37-38, 41-42, 47, 52-53, 66, 68, 73, 78-79, 83, 86-87, 91-92, 96, 103
Seemingly incurable diseases, 2, 31, 43, 100
Shivering, 40
Skin diseases, 52
Smoking, 20, 33, 84, 90
Stuttering, 93

T,U

Teething, 94
Throat, 3, 8, 20, 43, 57, 64, 91, 94
Tinnitus, 65, 94
Trigeminal neuralgia, 83, 94-95
Tuberculosis, 39, 86, 95
Ulcers, 73, 75, 91-92, 95-96

V,W

Vaginal discharge, 96
Varicose veins, 96-97
Warts, 62, 97
Water-treading, 65, 78, 97-98
Water treatments, 33, 65-66, 68, 78, 97
Water veins, 34, 43, 100

IMPORTANT RECIPES FOR THE TOTAL CANCER TREATMENT:

Breuss juice mixture .... *pg* 28
Sage tea .... *pg* 29
Kidney tea .... *pg* 30
Cranesbill tea .... *pg* 31
Onion broth .... *pg* 36

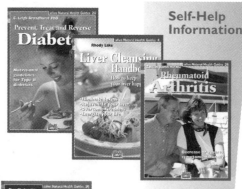
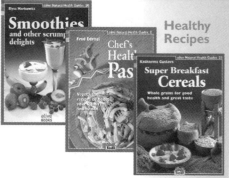
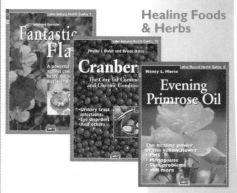
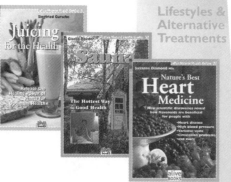